ILLUSTRATED TEXTBOOK OF

GYNAECOLOGY

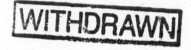

A slide Atlas of *Illustrated Textbook of Gynaecology* based on
the contents of this book, is available. In the slide atlas format,
the material is split into volumes, each of which is presented in a
binder together with numbered 35mm slides of each illustration.
Each slide atlas volume also contains a list of abbreviated slide
captions for easy reference when using the slides. Further
information can be obtained from:

Gower Medical Publishing
Middlesex House
34-42 Cleveland Street
London W1P 5FB

Gower Medical Publishing
101 5th Avenue
New York, NY. 1003
USA

ILLUSTRATED TEXTBOOK OF

GYNAECOLOGY

V R TINDALL MSc MD FRCSE FRCOG

Professor of Obstetrics and Gynaecology
based at St Mary's Hospital
University of Manchester

SHARON OATES MB ChB MRCOG

Lecturer, Honorary Senior Registrar
Department of Obstetrics and Gynaecology
St Mary's Hospital, Manchester

SILVIA RIMMER MB ChB FFR DMRD

Consultant Radiologist
St Mary's Hospital, Manchester

ARB SMITH MD MRCOG

Consultant Obstetrician and Gynaecologist
St Mary's Hospital, Manchester

Gower Medical Publishing LONDON • NEW YORK

Distributed in the USA and Canada by:
J B Lippincott Company
East Washington Square
Philadelphia
PA 19105
USA

Distributed in the UK and Continental Europe by:
Gower Medical Publishing
Middlesex House
34-42 Cleveland Street
London W1P 5FB

Distributed in Australia and New Zealand by:
Harper and Row (Australia) Pty Ltd
PO Box 226
Artarmon
NSW 2064
AUSTRALIA

Distributed in Southeast Asia, Hong Kong, India
and Pakistan by:
Harper and Row (Asia) Pte Ltd
37 Jalan Pemimpin 02-01
Singapore 2057

Distributed in Japan by:
Nankodo Co Ltd
42-6 Hongo 3-chome
Bunkyo-ku
Tokyo 113

Project Managers:	Suzanne Evans Robert Whittle
Design:	Louise Bond Balvir Koura
Illustration:	Marion Tasker Dereck Johnson Lee Smith Sue Tyler
Paste-up artist:	Ruth Miles
Production:	Susan Bishop Adam Phillips
Publisher:	Fiona Foley

Originated in Hong Kong by Bright Arts (HK) Ltd.
Typesetting by Ampersand Typesetters Ltd,
Bournemouth.
Text set in Sabon; captions and figures set in Univers.
Printed in Hong Kong, produced by Mandarin.

British Library Cataloguing in Publication Data:
Tindall, Victor
Illustrated textbook of gynaecology.
1. Gynaecology
I. Tindall, V. R. (Victor Ronald) *1928*-
618.1
ISBN 0-397-44728-0

Library of Congress Cataloging-in-Publication Data
Illustrated textbook of gynaecology/V.R. Tindall...
[et al.].
Companion volume to: Illustrated textbook of
Obstetrics
Includes index.
1. Gynecology. I. Tindall, V.R. II. Illustrated textbook of
obstetrics.
[DNLM 1. Gynecology. WP 100 I283]
RG101.I45 1991
618.1--dc20

Preface

When it was suggested that there should be a companion volume in Gynaecology to *Illustrated Textbook of Obstetrics*, I thought this would be a relatively simple task, but it was not. The notes produced in the past for our students in Manchester were thought to be an ideal basis for the text, and the illustrations and flow charts would therefore follow quite easily. However, this was not the case, and the gestation period has therefore been much longer than intended. The only consolation is that it has been slightly shorter than the gestation period of the first edition of its companion volume.

Having been told at an early stage in one's postgraduate career that in answering examination questions a diagram, if it is correct, is worth half a page of writing, I should have appreciated how difficult it would be to produce this book. I certainly hope that in the majority of figures we have provided some confirmation that it saved words. In order to keep to an extended deadline, I involved some of my Manchester colleagues: my Lecturer, albeit on a temporary basis, Dr Sharon Oates who, like myself, is a graduate from Liverpool with all its tradition of undergraduate teaching; Dr Sylvia Rimmer, a Consultant Radiologist who graduated from Manchester and who provides all the Obstetricians and Gynaecologists at Saint Mary's Hospital with such an excellent service, for the chapter on Gynaecological Imaging; and Dr Tony Smith, another true Mancunian who, having graduated and trained in Manchester before moving to Sheffield as Lecturer, has recently returned as Consultant at Saint Mary's Hospital.

We have all endeavoured to make this book appropriate for the present-day undergraduate who spends only about eight weeks doing Obstetrics and Gynaecology. It is hoped that this book will provide the stimulus for easy reading, learning and, when appropriate, revision. If it does then we will have achieved our principal aim. It could, however, not have been achieved without the help of the talented artist, Marion Tasker, who has made so much out of the varied and often poor quality material we presented to her, and Mrs Eileen Silver who, despite many other commitments, managed to produce the text.

V R TINDALL
Manchester 1991

Contents

1 | The Seven Ages of Woman

In *As You Like It* Shakespeare considers that –

'one man in his time plays many parts, his acts being seven stages'.

If, by analogy, one considers women and their phases of life then they have seven principle stages of varying duration. They include:

SEVEN AGES OF WOMAN	
1 an intrauterine phase	5 a reproductive era
2 infancy	6 the climacteric phase
3 childhood	7 the geriatric era
4 adolescence	

This last phase is aptly qualified by Shakespeare as a phase of 'second childishness, and mere oblivion, sans teeth, sans eyes, sans taste, sans everything'.

Whilst there is an inevitable overlap of gynaecological symptoms and conditions in some of these groups there are also problems which are only encountered in one of the seven eras of a woman's life. A knowledge of the normal structure and physiology of the female reproductive system and any abnormality which may occur throughout life is of benefit to all medical students. It is not always appreciated how much influence obstetrical practice and trauma exerts on gynaecology.

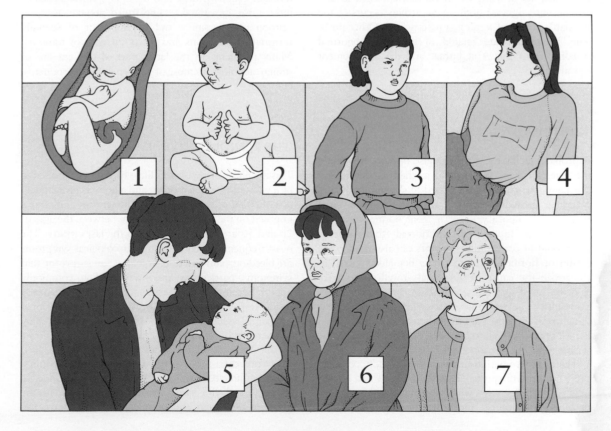

INTRAUTERINE LIFE

It is during this phase that normal (or abnormal) development of the genital tract and sexual determination occurs. For example, it is well known that the habits of the mother, such as smoking, alcohol and drug addiction, can determine the subsequent growth pattern of her child. Other drugs taken by the mother during pregnancy may affect their daughters in later life. Oestrogens, which at one time were given to help establish or retain a pregnancy, were subsequently found to be associated with an unusual type of clear cell carcinoma of the vagina or cervix, the malignancy developing when the daughter was a teenager or in her early twenties.

INFANCY

There may be doubt about the sex of an infant at, or shortly after, birth. The early recognition of a defect, such as the adrenogenital syndrome, allows one to select the proper age at which to correct it. Many basic defects remain unrecognised until sexual activity occurs or the woman's potential fertility is investigated. Other problems in infancy are related to infection, abnormal bleeding from the genital tract and the development of tumours.

CHILDHOOD

A problem facing the gynaecologist, or more frequently the paediatrician, is whether a child is developing normally particularly with regard to skeletal, body and glandular growth. It may be necessary to establish if there is a temporary or permanent hormonal cause. However, it must be remembered that genetic, nutritional or constitutional factors can also modify the action of hormones. In fact it is not always easy to categorize the cause of abnormal growth since there may be an associated gonadal or chromosomal abnormality. The principle concern of parents is their daughter's growth pattern, whereas with the child herself it is often related to breast development, as she wishes to be like her contemporaries.

There are two periods in infancy and childhood when there are growth spurts. (1) After the birth and for the next two or three years when a great increase in skeletal development occurs, and then a slower and more orderly pattern follows until the gonadotrophins act. (2) At about the time of puberty there is another growth spurt. If a child is too fat or too thin, too tall or too short, then the parents become anxious. There may be precocious development in one or more areas, or an inhibiting influence may prevent normal development. The detection of the underlying cause is important as some defects can be corrected.

ADOLESCENCE

This is the phase of development from childhood to adulthood in the years between puberty and the attainment of maturity. In women this is on average from 12 to 20 years, although it does depend largely on socio-economic and environmental factors. The principle gynaecological problems in this phase are related to puberty and the adjustment to menstruation, symptoms associated with menstruation or dysfunctional bleeding. This is an era of sexual awareness with particular anxieties about secondary sex characteristics. Problems may also arise as a consequence of intercourse, unwanted or unplanned pregnancies, prevention of pregnancy and development of sexually transmitted infections and the occurrence of tumours. Many problems in the latter part of this era are of similar aetiology to those of women in the reproductive era.

THE REPRODUCTIVE ERA

This is a phase of a woman's life where she is expected to be a worker, a lover, a mother, and a housekeeper, and all too often all at the same time. The stresses and strains imposed on the present day woman between the ages of 20 and 50 are far greater than in the last century. The most frequently encountered gynaecological symptoms are bleeding, pain and discharge. It is not surprising that symptoms, particularly abnormal bleeding, commonly appear because of their association with a pregnancy inside or outside the uterus. Infections and vaginal discharges assume increasing importance as they may interfere with conception. Treatment will concentrate on the symptoms and overcoming any factor which might prevent a future pregnancy. If surgery is required it will be directed towards conservation of reproductive capacity and the same principle will apply in the presence of benign and premalignant conditions. Endocrinological problems are, in general, related to secondary amenorrhoea and subfertility. Indeed, many gynaecological problems are related to the desire to conceive, or the wish to avoid pregnancy on a temporary or permanent basis so that the family of the desired size and at the right time is achieved. Although, whilst our ability to diagnose and treat infertile women has improved considerably over the past two decades, advance with regard to male infertility has been negligible.

Nowadays, every woman anticipates that once conception occurs it will be followed by the production of a normal and healthy infant, unfortunately for one reason or another this outcome is not always attainable at the present time.

THE CLIMACTERIC PHASE

This occurs about a year or so after the menopause and is associated with cessation of ovarian function. It is also the time in a woman's life when her children are leaving home and her husband or partner is reaching, or is at the peak of his chosen career. The adaptation to changing circumstances and hormonal deficiency in the majority of women can produce a multitude of gynaecological symptoms such as hot flushes and insomnia. The loss of ovarian function is also associated with symptoms related to the gastrointestinal tract and urinary tract, as well as relaxation of the pelvic floor tissues and prolapse. It is also the time when malignancies of the reproductive organs are increasing in incidence and any bleeding after the menopause should be considered due to a malignancy until proven otherwise.

Approximately a quarter to one third of a woman's life span is likely to continue after the menopause and because of this the role of hormone replacement therapy has become a major issue in the developed countries of the world.

THE GERIATRIC PHASE

The process of ageing varies from one person to another and it is important to consider the woman's physiological age rather than her chronological age. If an elderly woman has a gynaecological problem, then it has to be determined what can realistically be achieved and to what extent one can overcome her difficulties. If surgery is considered in a woman of advanced years the aim is to make her comfortable, useful and happy as long as her life continues.

Common gynaecological problems in elderly women are related to the damage of tissues during previous labours and in particular are referrable to the bladder and urinary tract. The majority of gynaecological symptoms in women over 65 are related to postmenopausal bleeding, genital prolapse, alterations in normal bladder function and infections. Another common complaint is the discovery of a mass in the vulva, vagina, abdomen or breast.

In this last phase of life it is essential that there is adequate pre-operative assessment and preparation if surgery is considered necessary, and if so, particular attention must be paid to post-operative care and rehabilitation.

In all phases of a woman's life it is important to allow the woman (or her parents) to explain the problem, for any pre-conceived thoughts about the diagnosis are likely to be followed by the wrong treatment. It should also be remembered that often no specific therapy is required other than an explanation of the diagnosis and reassurance that there is no serious disease present. It is not surprising that with the multitude of roles a woman has to adapt to, some disturbance of function occurs from time to time in any age group. Despite this women survive on average four to five years longer than men, thus supporting the view that, biologically, women are the stronger sex.

INTRODUCTION

The development and growth of a woman is associated with major changes in the physiological functions of various organs and their ability to adapt to these changes. All systems are affected, but whilst we have knowledge of the events that occur, it is not always possible to predict how an individual girl or woman will react to the development of sexual characteristics, reproduction or the menopause. Indeed, it is at these times that the skills of the medical attendants may be directed towards reassurance rather than their diagnostic or therapeutic skills.

DEVELOPMENT AND GROWTH

The urinary tract and genital organs develop in close association. Any anomaly in one is often accompanied

LANDMARKS IN EARLY DEVELOPMENT	
Week 1	fertilization in the Fallopian tube to implantation in the uterus; genetic sex determined
Week 2	bilaminar germ disc embryo
Week 3	formation of third embryonic layer
Weeks 4–8	beginning of development of all major internal and external organs and organ systems (major congenital malformations occur if embryo is exposed to teratogens)
Weeks 7–8	development of ovary
Weeks 10–12	formation of upper and lower genital tract and urinary tract

Fig. 2.1 Landmarks in early development.

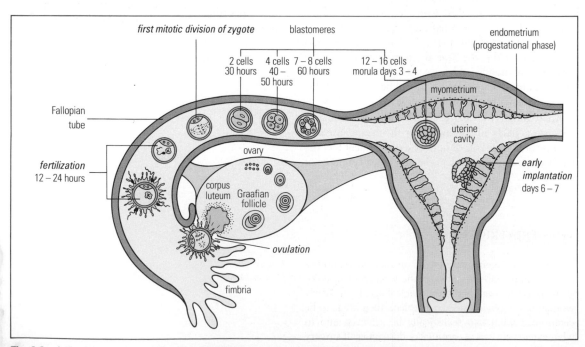

Fig. 2.2 A diagrammatic representation of fertilization and early implantation of the conceptus into the uterus.

by anomalies in the other. It is therefore useful to consider them together.

The principal landmarks in development from conception, implantation and embryogenesis are detailed in Figs 2.1 and 2.2. It should be appreciated that with the rapid development from one cell to millions of cells in the space of a few weeks internal and external influences can interfere with normal developmental processes. This may result in some abnormality or defect in the embryo, which may cause failure of development or even death.

The sex of the embryo is determined by the sperm that fertilizes the ovum. The process of normal gametogenesis is illustrated in Fig. 2.3. Normally an individual has 46 chromosomes of which 44 are autosomes and 2 are sex chromosomes. The sex chromosomes are designated X or Y. A configuration of 44 plus XX is female, whilst that of 44 plus XY is male.

Before the seventh week of embryonic life the gonads of both sexes are undifferentiated and identical in appearance and all human embryos are potentially bisexual initially. The combination of sex chromosomes at fertilization determines the gonadal type and this determines the subsequent sexual differentiation seen in the genital ducts and external genitalia. If a Y chromosome is present the embryo is male, because the Y chromosome has a testis determining effect on the medulla of the undifferentiated gonad. In the absence of a Y chromosome an ovary forms. The number of X chromosomes present is unimportant in sex determination although two X chromosomes are necessary for complete ovarian development. Loss of an X chromosome causes ovarian dysgenesis (Turner's syndrome). This results from non-disjunction of the sex chromosomes at gametogenesis and is discussed further later in the chapter.

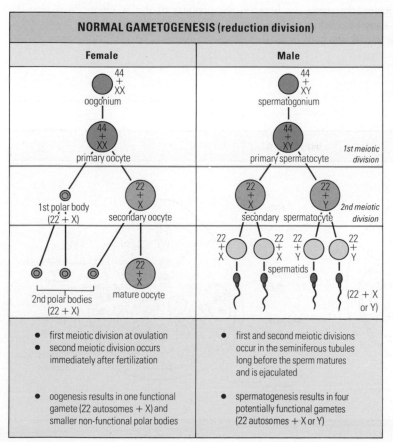

Fig. 2.3 The fundamental difference between gametogenesis in the male and female is the unequal duration of meiosis in the two sexes. In the female the process begun during fetal life is suspended until puberty. In males meiosis occurs within several days.

The gonads, the testes or ovaries, are formed from two types of cells, the primordial germ cells and the nutrient supporting cells (the follicular cells of the ovary; the Sertoli cells of the testis). The primordial germ cells on each side migrate by an amoeboid movement along the dorsal mesentery of the hindgut during the fifth week and reach the lumbar region of the developing embryo, the future genital ridges (Fig. 2.4). If the cells fail to reach the ridges the gonads do not develop and gonadal dysgenesis occurs.

In the sixth week the primordial germ cells invade the genital ridges and are incorporated into the primary sex cords which proliferate and grow from the coelomic epithelium into the underlying mesenchyme. The gonad at this stage has the same appearance in the male and female and this indifferent gonad has an outer cortex and an inner medulla. In female embryos the cortex forms the ovary and the medulla regresses.

The ovary is identifiable by the tenth week of embryonic life. During fetal life the primordial follicles (oogonia) are distributed in a connective tissue stroma. Their number is limited and about a quarter to two million are present at birth. Each contains the reproductive cell, an oocyte, at a primary stage of development with 46 chromosomes. Of the initial stock of primordial follicles, only about 300 develop between puberty and the menopause to produce fertilizable ova. Active mitosis of oogonia occurs during fetal life and none are formed after birth. The primary oocyte surrounded by one or two layers of follicular cells is called a primary follicle and most are quiescent until puberty.

The primitive genital tract

The genital tracts are similar in male and female embryos until the seventh week and consist of two paramesonephric (Mullerian) ducts and two mesonephric (Wolffian) ducts (Fig. 2.5). The Mullerian ducts cross in front of the Wolffian ducts and run alongside them. The terminal parts of the Mullerian ducts fuse to form a single median duct (uterovaginal canal), which ends blindly at the posterior surface of the urogenital sinus. The blind ending projects into the dorsal wall of the sinus to create the Mullerian tubule, which is located between the opening of the Wolffian ducts into the urogenital sinus.

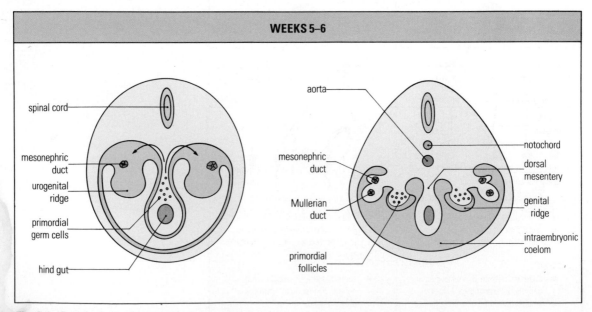

WEEKS 5–6

Fig. 2.4 Development of the gonad.

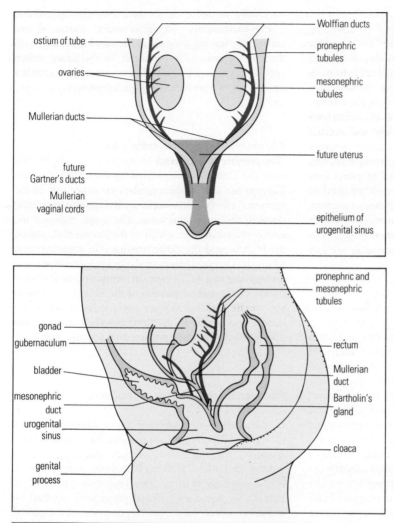

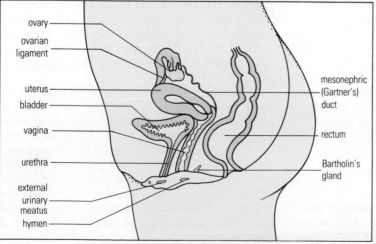

Fig. 2.5 Development of the internal genitalia. Diagram of the Mullerian and Wolffian systems, front view (upper). The undifferentiated genital tract in lateral view (middle). Adult female genitalia (lower). The Mullerian ducts have fused to form the uterus and vagina.

Development of the internal genitalia

In females, the mesonephric (Wolffian) ducts regress and the paramesonephric (Mullerian) ducts develop to form the female genital tract. The cranial unfused parts of the Mullerian ducts form the uterine (Fallopian) tubes and the caudal fused parts form a single median uterovaginal canal which gives rise to the epithelium and glands of the uterus (Fig. 2.5). The endometrial stroma and myometrium develops from the adjacent mesenchyme. The fusion of the caudal parts commences caudally and progresses up to the future Fallopian tubes. The median septum disappears by the end of the first trimester. Fusion of the Mullerian ducts brings together two peritoneal compartments, the uterorectal pouch (Pouch of Douglas) and the uterovesical pouch. The remnants of the two Wolffian ducts persist as vestigial structures (Gartner's ducts).

Formation of the vagina

The terminal end of the primitive uterovaginal canal reaches the posterior wall of the urogenital sinus and forms a tubercle. The posterior wall of the urogenital sinus thickens opposite the tubercle and together they form the vaginal epithelial plate. From this plate, two solid evaginations, the sinovaginal bulbs, grow and encircle the caudal end of the primitive uterovaginal canal. Canalization of the vaginal plate begins in the eleventh week and proceeds from the caudal to cranial end forming the vagina with the peripheral cells remaining as the vaginal epithelium. Canalization is complete by the fifth intrauterine month. The sinovaginal bulbs surround the cervix of the uterus to form the fornices of the vagina. Thus the vagina is of endodermal origin, derived from the wall of the urogenital sinus. The paramesonephric ducts form the body and cervix of the uterus. The vaginal lumen remains separated from the urogenital sinus until late fetal life by a membrane which is situated just above the hymen. Buds from the urethra grow into the mesenchyme and form the urethral glands and the paraurethral glands (of Skene). Outgrowths from the urogenital sinus form the greater (Bartholin's) vestibular glands.

The upper portion of the genital tract

The cranial opening of the paramesonephric duct, which is open to the peritoneal cavity develops into the fimbriae of the uterine tube. The Fallopian tube eventually moves caudally and becomes horizontal.

The mesonephric (Wolffian) ducts regress almost completely, leaving only a short segment connected with the mesonephric tubes adjacent to the ovary which persists as the epoophoron. Other mesonephric tubules caudal to the ovary form the paroophoron.

The lower portion of the genital tract

The urogenital sinus and anorectal canal are formed from the cloaca and separated by the urorectal sinus. Three zones can be distinguished on either side of the openings of the mesonephric and paramesonephric ducts in the urogenital sinus. The upper region is the vesicourethral section which in the female gives rise to the bladder and the entire urethra. The middle region forms the vaginal opening and, the lowest section is the area surrounded by the external genital organs. Differentiation of the genital portion of the urogenital sinus in the female follows that of the urogenital excretory system and begins in the third month, paralleling the formation of the vagina and external organs.

Development of the female external genital organs

In the absence of androgens the indifferent external genitalia will undergo feminization. The cloacal membrane by the third week is very extensive, and its anterior end is level with the base of the umbilical cord. It is at this stage that the cloacal membrane is bordered laterally by two mesenchymal projections, covered by ectoderm, which are the paired precursors of the genital tubercle. The anterior end of the cloacal membrane retracts from the base of the umbilical cord, permitting formation of the anterior body wall below the umbilicus, and the paired precursors of the genital tubercle come together in the midline to form the genital tubercle (Fig. 2.6).

The cloacal fold, which surrounds the cloacal membrane prolongs the genital tubercle. New swellings appear on either side of the cloacal folds, and surround the genital tubercle and the cloacal folds. By the seventh week, the cloacal membrane is divided anteriorly into the urogenital membrane and posteriorly the anal membrane is separated by the perineal body (perineum).

Differentiation of the external genitalia takes place during the third intrauterine month and closely follows the pattern of the primitive structures. The genital tubercle elongates only slightly and forms the clitoris, where erectile tissue develops. The urogenital sinus remains open with the urethra opening anteriorly and the vagina posteriorly, within the interior of the vestibule portion of the sinus. The vestibule which is bordered laterally by the genital folds, becomes the labia minora. The genital swellings largely remain unfused and form the labia majora. Although they unite posteriorly to form the posterior labial commensure and anteriorly to form the mons pubis.

The urinary system

The urinary system develops in the mesoderm on the posterior wall of the coelomic cavity. The three embryological stages are; the pronephros, the mesonephros and the metanephros.

The pronephros is a transient structure which exists for only a few weeks during development.

The mesonephros is comprised of a series of tubules which extend from the lower thoracic and upper lumbar region, and are joined to the longitudinal mesonephric, or Wolffian duct. The mesonephric duct develops a group of temporarily active tubular cells which act as an excretory organ for a few weeks. The definitive kidney develops from the metanephros system.

The metanephros, or permanent kidney, develops from two sources; the ureteric bud on the mesonephric duct, which forms the drainage system, and the metanephric cap, which forms the substance of the adult kidney. The ureteric bud grows upwards to meet the metanephric cap. The bud forms the ureter, renal pelvis and distal parts of the collecting tubules. The cap forms the glomerular capsules, convoluted tubules and loops of Henlé.

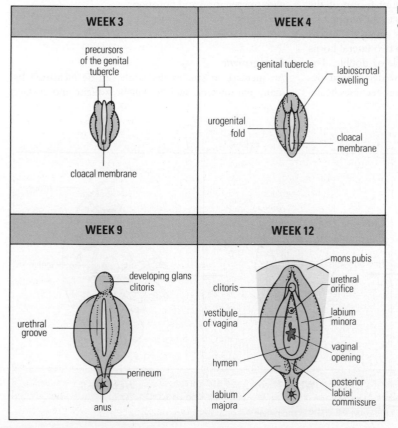

Fig. 2.6 Development of the female external genitalia.

9

Initially, the metanephros is entirely a pelvic organ, lying over the upper sacral segments and receiving its blood supply from the aorta. The apparent ascent of the kidneys in the abdomen is actually due to rapid caudal growth, drawing the kidneys upwards, so that in adult life they are at the level of the high lumbar vertebrae (Fig. 2.7). Congenital abnormalities of the urinary tract, such as renal fusion, hypoplasia and dysplasia are not uncommon.

The trigone and posterior prostatic urethra develop from the mesonephric ducts. The remainder of the bladder and urethra develop from the urogenital sinus. From the upper end of the fundus of the bladder, the urachus, a remnant of the allantois runs to the umbilicus. This is often hollow and accompanies the obliterated umbilical vessels. This, in turn, represents the anterior portion of the early cloaca, a common ectodermal invagination into which the alimentary and urinary systems open.

Uterovaginal malformations

As a result of partial or total failure of fusion of the terminal portions of the Mullerian ducts, formation of a double uterus, cervix and vagina may occur, the uterus can become more or less divided into two lateral horns (bicollis) and the cervix may be single or double. The uterus may be incomplete with a wedge-shaped depression at the fundus so that the uterus becomes heart-shaped, or the uterus can be absent altogether. These and other possible malformations, are illustrated in Fig. 2.8.

Partial or total atresia of the terminal portion of one or both Mullerian ducts may produce unilateral atresia or a rudimentary horn. Alternatively partial bilateral atresia with atresia of the cervix or the vagina may result, or the vagina may be absent.

Development of the embryo and fetus

After fertilization the blastocyst grows rapidly in the uterus. It is conventionally called an embryo after organ formation starts (at two weeks), and a fetus after organogenesis is complete (at ten weeks). In combination with the placenta, the fetus creates a *milieu interieur*, which permits its own survival and, in doing so, alters major maternal physiological processes. One of the major differences between intra- and extrauterine life lies in the role of the placenta; this, rather than the lungs and the alimentary tract, provides the fetus with oxygenation and nutrition.

Fetal growth

An increase in size in the adult can be measured by many parameters, such as height, weight and surface

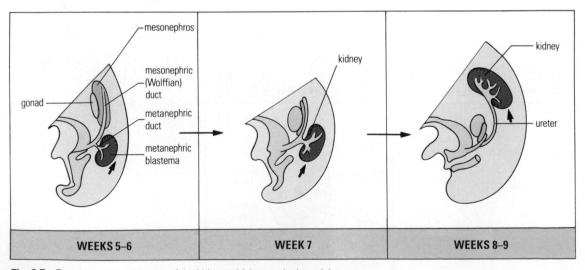

Fig. 2.7 Development and ascent of the kidney which starts in the pelvis.

area of various dimensions, in unit time. The fetus *in utero*, however, can only be measured by non-invasive methods using longitudinal ultrasound.

Fetal growth expressed in weight gain per week, is slow and gradual until twenty weeks. The rate of growth then becomes faster between 24 and 34 weeks of gestation. Growth, particularly of the head, is the most notable feature of fetal physiology. Hence the fetal head is much larger in relation to its body and limbs than that of an older child or adult (Fig. 2.9). The growth rate is faster than that of the rest of the body, due to the preferential supply of blood to the cephalic end of the fetus.

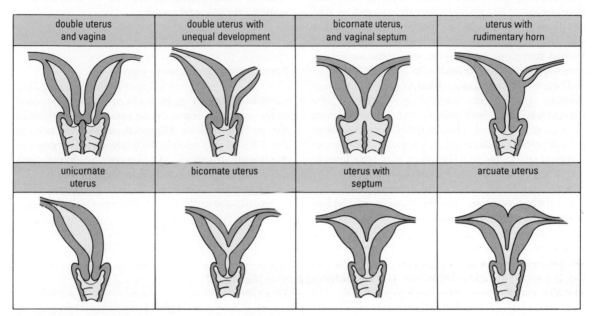

| double uterus and vagina | double uterus with unequal development | bicornate uterus, and vaginal septum | uterus with rudimentary horn |
| unicornate uterus | bicornate uterus | uterus with septum | arcuate uterus |

Fig. 2.8   Diagram to show various uterine malformations.

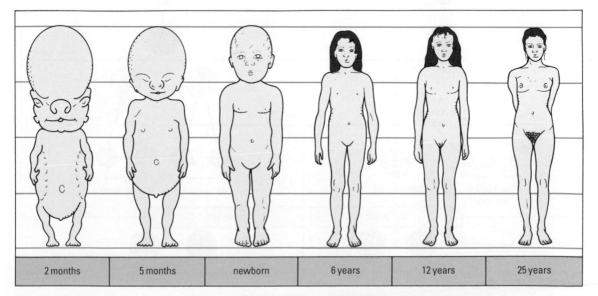

| 2 months | 5 months | newborn | 6 years | 12 years | 25 years |

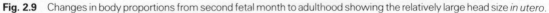

Fig. 2.9   Changes in body proportions from second fetal month to adulthood showing the relatively large head size *in utero*.

Extrauterine growth and development

The early development of a newborn infant depends on parental care and nourishment for survival. The period of infancy which comprises the first two years of life and early childhood is associated with well established landmarks of achievement. Childhood problems are largely concerned with somatic growth and development. The only time the gynaecologist or paediatrician is likely to be involved is if the parents feel that their daughter is not following their views of normal growth or development, or if there are specific symptoms which require attention.

The principle problems related to growth are either delayed development, particularly related to the changes associated with puberty and the development of secondary sexual characteristics, or precocious puberty, which is discussed in Chapter 5. The gynaecological conditions which produce local symptoms in a young child are related to trauma and infection. The exposed position of the vulva in a child makes it particularly vulnerable, and the majority of children between the ages of two and eight who have problems

have vulvo-vaginal discharge. In many cases, the cause is related to inadequate hygiene. There are also a few dermatological conditions which may occur in association with a co-existing vulvo-vaginitis, eg. condylomata, or others such as lichen sclerosis, or psoriasis, that manifest themselves in childhood. The majority of injuries are usually caused by an accident or fall on a blunt or sharp object, but may be self-inflicted or a consequence of sexual assault.

Sexual anomalies of genetic origin

Gonadal dysgenesis can be due to a failure of disjunction of the sex chromosomes during gametogenesis in one of the parents. This is illustrated diagrammatically in Fig. 2.10 and may result in the following conditions:
• Ovarian dysgenesis XO (Turner's syndrome) with female morphology and a karyotype of only one sex chromosome which is X (Fig. 2.11). However, mosaics also exist.

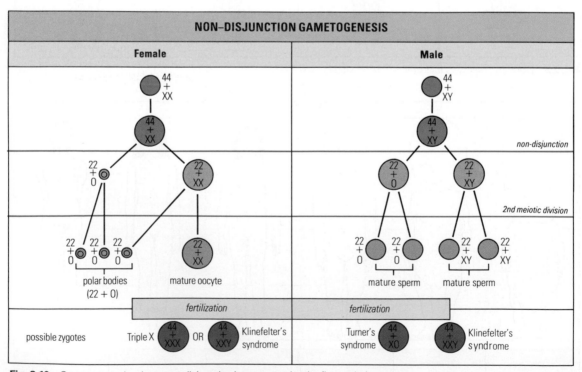

Fig. 2.10 Gametogenesis where non-disjunction has occurred at the first meiotic division (cf. Fig. 2.3). Triple X females have a normal appearance.

- Testicular dysgenesis (Klinefelter's syndrome) with male morphology and karyotype XXY (Fig. 2.11).
- Mixed gonadal dysgenesis, which is rare. A testis on one side and an undifferentiated gonad on the other. The internal genitalia are female, but male derivatives of the mesonephric ducts are present. The external genitalia range from normal female to intermediate normal male, but at puberty, neither breast development nor menstruation occurs. There are varying degrees of virilization and the condition is thought to be due to a combination of a defective Y chromosome and amounts of androgen present.
- Testicular feminization is also rare. The appearance is that of a normal female, despite the presence of testes and XY chromosomes. There is normal breast development at puberty, but no pubic hair and the vagina ends blindly. Other genitalia are absent or rudimentary. The testes are abdominal or inguinal, but may be in the labia majora. It is an extreme form of male pseudohermaphroditism, and is not a true intersex because the female external genitalia are normal. The testes develop and secrete androgens, but masculinization of the genitalia fails because

the 'indifferent' external genitalia are insensitive to androgens.

True hermaphroditism is exceedingly rare. It occurs as a consequence of failure of disjunction of sex chromosomes during the first cleavage mitosis of the egg and results in sex mosaics such as XY/XX or XY/XO.

The quantitative importance of the male (Y) chromosome explains the ultimate variations in androgenic effects, with varying degrees of the differentiation of the external genitalia and subtle variations in somatic morphology.

Sexual anomalies of hormonal origin

These are seen in people with normal genetic makeup. The primary and secondary sexual characteristics leading to pseudohermaphroditism are related to the effects of abnormal androgen secretion.

Male hermaphroditism is the result of an abnormal virilization of a female fetus that has normal ovaries and a 46 XX karyotype. Virilization may be of endogenous

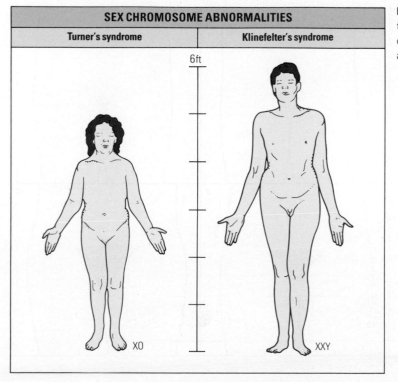

SEX CHROMOSOME ABNORMALITIES

Turner's syndrome	Klinefelter's syndrome

6ft

XO

XXY

Fig. 2.11 Diagrammatic comparison of the phenotypic appearance of two sex chromosome abnormalities: Turner's and Klinefelter's syndromes.

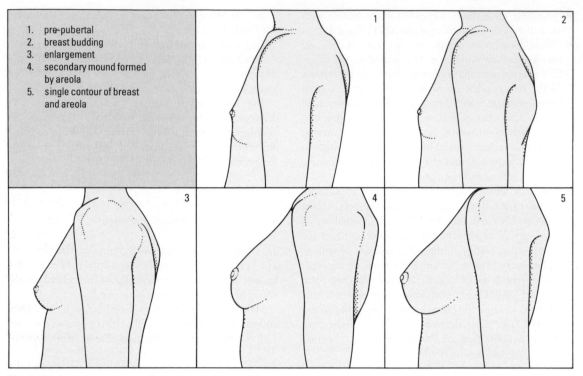

1. pre-pubertal
2. breast budding
3. enlargement
4. secondary mound formed by areola
5. single contour of breast and areola

Fig. 2.12 Breast development from pre-puberty to adulthood.

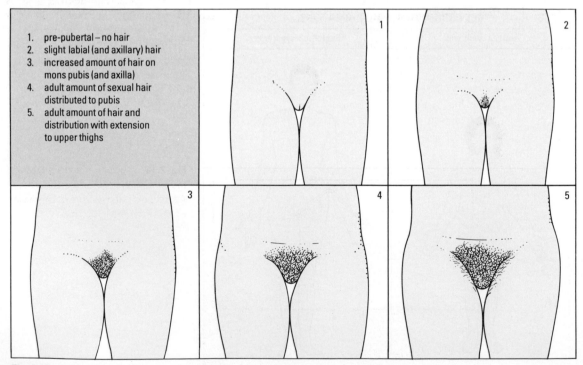

1. pre-pubertal – no hair
2. slight labial (and axillary) hair
3. increased amount of hair on mons pubis (and axilla)
4. adult amount of sexual hair distributed to pubis
5. adult amount of hair and distribution with extension to upper thighs

Fig. 2.13 Pubic hair growth.

origin, or due to excessive androgen secretion by the fetal adrenal, or of exogenous origin, related to administration of synthetic progesterone or anabolic steroids containing androgens. The paramesonephric system and differentiation of the external genitalia toward a male pattern, resulting in a peniform clitoris and a tendency to closure of the urogenital sinus.

PUBERTY

Puberty is the phase of life when the secondary sex characteristics develop and the gonads become active. In girls it is associated with the breasts increasing in size, the development of hair in the axilla and pubic regions. The ovaries, uterus and vagina also enlarge, but this is not as readily identifiable except for the onset of menstruation. Psychological changes occur as the girl matures towards adolescence and womanhood. The average age of these changes is variable and the dividing line between delayed puberty and precocious puberty is somewhat arbitrary and often related to the onset of menstruation.

Puberty is associated with a growth spurt followed by breast development, the appearance of pubic hair, changes in the external genitalia and the onset of menstruation. Breast development has been divided into specific phases, prepubertal, breast budding, enlargement, the formation of secondary mound formed by the areola and finally a single contour of breast and areola (Fig. 2.12). Pubic hair growth can also be divided into five stages, prepubertal (no hair), slight labial and axillary hair, increased amount of hair on mons pubis and in axilla, adult amount of sexual hair, but limited to pubis, adult amount and distribution of hair with extension to upper thigh (Fig. 2.13).

Significant variations in the time sequence of events are common without there being any specific cause (Fig. 2.14). Within three to four years of its onset sexual development will be completed and girls usually reach their final height about 2 years after the onset of menstruation (menarche). Delayed puberty is generally accepted as delayed when the breast and/or hair development have not taken place by the age of 13–14 years. Precocious puberty is generally accepted when the secondary sex characteristics develop before the age of eight. The average age of menarche is 12–13 years (±2–3 years). It is considered that body composition is a factor in determining the onset of puberty and menstruation. Individuals who are moderately obese, 20–30% above the ideal body weight, usually have an early menarche. Malnutrition delays the onset of puberty and it may occur in well nourished individuals if they undergo routine strenuous exercise before the menarche.

Before puberty circulating levels of follicle stimulating hormone (FSH) and luteinizing hormone (LH) are low (ratio of FSH/LH greater than 1) because the hypothalamus is very sensitive to the negative feedback of low levels of circulating oestrogen. It is generally accepted that the hormonal changes characteristic of puberty result from an increase in sensitivity of the hypothalamic centre which regulates gonadotrophin secretion. The precise mechanism for this change in sensitivity and for the increase in the pulses of gonadotrophin releasing hormone (GnRh) is unknown. It seems likely that several brain neurotransmitters play a part. There is also an associated

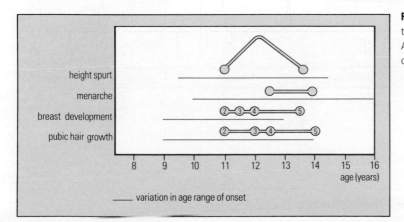

Fig. 2.14 A graphical representation of the principle changes at the menarche. Also shown is the variation of age range of onset commonly observed.

maturation or altered biological response of other organs or tissues to the gonadotrophic and steroid hormones.

In the male the testis has the power of spermatogenesis from puberty until death, new spermatozoa developing constantly. The ovary, however, does not produce ova in this fashion. The number of oocytes is maximal before birth. One estimate puts the figures as follows:

2 months	600,000 germ cells
5 months	7,000,000 germ cells
Birth	2,000,000 germ cells

The management of delayed and precocious puberty is dealt with in Chapter 6, Gynaecological conditions.

Menstrual cycle

Menstruation is a visible manifestation of the cyclical secretion of hormones occurring in a well-integrated manner, involving several organs (Fig. 2.15). The clinical arbitrary nomenclature, whereby the onset of menstruation is termed day one of the cycle, does not correlate with the hormone cycles, since menstruation represents the end of the hormone cycle.

The cycle commences with the release of gonadotrophin releasing hormone (GnRh) from the hypothalamus (Fig. 2.16). GnRh is secreted in a pulsatile manner and the amplitude and frequency of the pulse varies throughout the menstrual cycle. The frequency being more rapid in the follicular phase and slower in the luteal phase. GnRh stimulates both the synthesis and

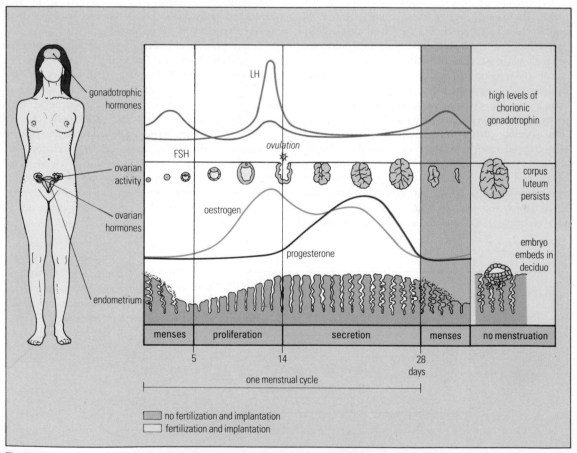

Fig. 2.15 The menstrual cycle: the effects of the pituitary hormones on the ovary, ovarian hormone production and endometrium.

the secretion of luteinizing hormone (LH) and follicle stimulating hormone (FSH) from the same cells in the anterior lobe of the pituitary gland. GnRh brings about the release of FSH which acts on the ovary to bring about the early maturation of several follicles. One of the follicles however, quickly outstrips the remainder which become atretic. FSH stimulates follicular growth by increasing both FSH and LH receptor sites in granulosa cells. This action is enhanced by oestrogen.

The ripening follicle produces oestrogens from the membrana glomerulosa and theca interna. The oestrogens have specific effects on various target organs, as follows:

(i) A negative feedback to suppress FSH release.

(ii) A positive feedback to produce GnRh and LH release from the anterior pituitary.

LH brings about rupture of the follicle releasing the ovum and the follicle then develops into a corpus luteum. LH also stimulates synthesis of prostaglandins which are involved in luteinization of the follicle and production of progesterone. Prostaglandins have an important function in the process of rupture of the follicle. The follicular content of prostaglandin increases markedly at the time of the mid-cycle LH surge, shortly before ovulation occurs. The corpus luteum produces progesterone and oestrogens. Due to the suppression of FSH release the oestrogen level begins to fall until the corpus luteum develops and produces more, thus oestrogen secretion is biphasic.

The rising levels of oestrogen and progesterone have an inhibitory effect on GnRh altering the frequency and amplitude of the GnRh pulses. This affects the release of LH which falls with consequent degeneration of the corpus luteum unless fertilization occurs. Following this there is a fall in oestrogen and progesterone levels and less negative feedback. As the oestrogen and progesterone levels decrease the pattern of GnRh release changes again and another cycle commences.

Endometrial cycle

The endometrium is one of the main target organs responding to hormonal stimulation (see Fig. 2.15). At the end of menstruation, the basal layer of the endometrium remains, the glands broken. The surface is rapidly epithelialized and is intact within two to three days. New vessels grow from the stumps of the old. Glands and stroma reform, at this stage the glands are small, lined by cuboidal epithelium and lie parallel to the endometrial surface. Under oestrogen stimulation rapid

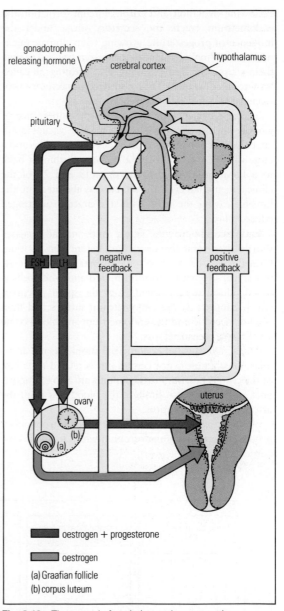

Fig. 2.16 The control of ovulation and menstruation showing the positive and negative oestrogen and progesterone feedback mechanism.

proliferation occurs, the glands become perpendicular to the surface as they grow. Whereas at the end of menstruation the endometrium is only 1mm thick, it is 3mm thick some ten days later. This is the proliferative phase.

17

Following ovulation and corpus luteum formation the endometrium enters the secretory phase under the influence of progesterone, growing to an ultimate thickness of 5 to 7mm. The glands increase in size and change their shape, the walls folding and creating so-called 'saw-toothed' glands. They also become secretory producing a secretion rich in glycogen.

The first evidence of secretion is the appearance of globules below the nucleus (subnuclear vacuolation), later the secretion moves to the sides of the nucleus and a large vacuole forms above the nucleus, flushing it back to a basal position. Between days 19 and 22 of the clinical menstrual cycle the secretion is liberated into the lumen, leaving the cells with a characteristic fringed edge.

Endometrial growth slows and virtually ceases shortly after, some five or six days before menstruation. Over the next day or two some shrinkage is evident. At this stage, stromal infiltration by red and white cells is noted, blood is extravated from the spiral arterioles which contract as the endometrium shrinks and then become necrotic and the endometrium and blood come away as the menstrual loss.

The actual cause of endometrial shrinkage and arteriolar constriction is not certain but is related to failure of the corpus luteum. Prostaglandins are also of importance in this and also limiting the blood loss from the arterioles at menstruation.

Should conception occur the developing trophoblast produces chorionic gonadotrophin which maintains the corpus luteum.

Cervical cycle

In the first half of the cycle, under oestrogenic influence, the cervical glands proliferate and secrete a mucus, which becomes thinner, more profuse and stretchable towards ovulation. Threads of mucus up to 10cm long can be drawn at ovulation (Spinnbarkett phenomenon). The electrolyte composition of this mucus is such that on drying the crystals form a 'fern-like' pattern. So profuse is the mucus production at this stage that the patient may complain of excessive discharge. This mucus is easily penetrated by spermatozoa due to the spatial arrangement of glycoprotein micelles.

Following ovulation under progesterone influence, the mucus alters becoming thick, tenacious, small in amount, non-stretchable, impenetrable by spermatozoa and it loses the 'ferning' on drying. It forms a cervical 'plug' which, if pregnancy occurs, remains until labour when it comes away as the 'show'.

Vaginal cycle

Cyclical changes are readily seen in stained vaginal smears. In the unstimulated stage before follicular proliferation the cells are small with normal nuclei and stain blue. Oestrogen brings about marked changes, the cells become cornified with pyknotic nuclei, staining with pink eosin. Following ovulation the number of pyknotic cells falls, the desquamated cells showing rolled edges.

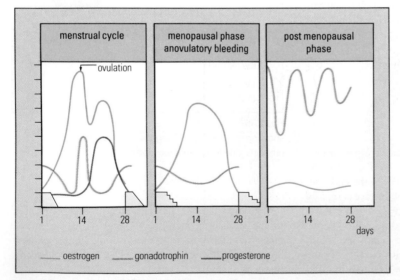

Fig. 2.17 Graphical representation of the gonadotrophin, oestrogen and progesterone levels in a normal menstrual cycle, an anovulatory cycle in the climacteric phase of life, and the post-menopause phase.

The ratio of pyknotic or cornified cells present on a smear, to the basal and intermediate cells is called the cornification index (CI) or karyopyknotic index (KPI) and is a guide to oestrogen activity, although used less frequently nowadays.

MENOPAUSE

Hormonal changes

The ageing of the ovary results in a gradual failure of response of the Graafian follicles to FSH stimulation and the secretion of oestrogen declines. As the level of oestrogen continues to fall, there is less inhibitory effect on the pituitary gland and thus some increase in FSH production occurs towards the end of this phase of life (climacteric). The feed-back effect of oestrogen on pituitary LH secretion is also partially removed. LH secretion as a consequence rises and the mid cycle peak becomes obliterated and anovulatory menstrual cycles occur. As ovarian function declines ovulation ceases completely. The absence of corpora lutea results in a reduction in progesterone secretion and eventually oestrogen levels become so low that menstrual bleeding becomes irregular and finally ceases (Fig. 2.17).

Menopausal symptoms are related to the falling oestrogen levels and the associated release of pituitary function. The rise in secretion of FSH may be associated with an increase in secretion of some of the pituitary trophic hormones. These include growth hormone, thyroid stimulating hormone (TSH) and adrenocorticotrophic hormone (ACTH). An increase in growth hormone levels after the menopause may result in obesity and mild acromegalic changes. There may also be an increase in atheromatous infiltration of the arterial system with a consequent rise in the incidence of coronary artery and other vascular diseases in postmenopausal women.

An increase in TSH in association with the imbalance between oestrogen and gonadotrophins often results in hot flushes and excessive sweating due to vasomotor instability. Emotional lability may also be related to the effect of TSH on its target organs. An increase in ACTH chiefly results in an excessive secretion of adrenocortical androgens which causes hirsutism, particularly noticeable on the face.

The failure of oestrogen production, apart from its indirect effects via the pituitary, is reflected primarily on the secondary sex organs. The breasts become smaller and lose their shape, the vulva and vaginal tissues become less vascular, and their epithelium more susceptible to injury and infection. Atrophic vaginitis with cracking, soreness and bleeding may occur. The ovary and uterus atrophy and the endometrium disappears completely.

The low oestrogen levels after menopause can also be associated with osteoporosis with resulting weakness of the weight bearing bones, particularly the vertebrae and the neck of the femur (Fig. 2.18).

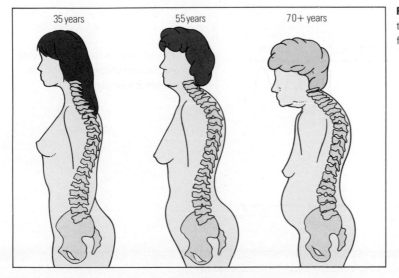

Fig. 2.18 The effects of the loss of tissue in the bone with loss of ovarian function.

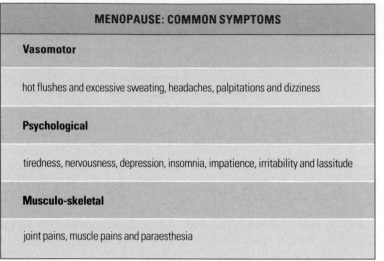

Fig. 2.19 Common symptoms of the menopause.

MENOPAUSE: COMMON SYMPTOMS
Vasomotor
hot flushes and excessive sweating, headaches, palpitations and dizziness
Psychological
tiredness, nervousness, depression, insomnia, impatience, irritability and lassitude
Musculo-skeletal
joint pains, muscle pains and paraesthesia

The majority of symptoms fall into three main groups and these are indicated in Fig. 2.19.

An explanation of the physiological changes, encouragement, non-hormonal therapy and support and/or appropriate hormone therapy will generally allow a woman to weather the disturbance of the menopause with a minimum of distress to herself and her family. The debate whether or not long-term hormone therapy is appropriate will be discussed later in Chapter 8.

INTRODUCTION

Before dealing with conditions caused by, or associated with, pathological changes one must have a detailed knowledge of the normal woman. From this one should be able to interpret the symptoms which may be caused by physiological or pathological changes in normal female homeostasis, and how these changes can be detected on examination. Finally, in this chapter screening for cancer in healthy, asymptomatic women is considered.

ANATOMY

The pelvic organs

In a lateral view of the pelvis and pelvic organs, the uterus usually lies in anteversion, so that the posterior fornix is deeper than the anterior fornix (Fig. 3.1). The anterior wall of the vagina lies against the base of the bladder and urethra.

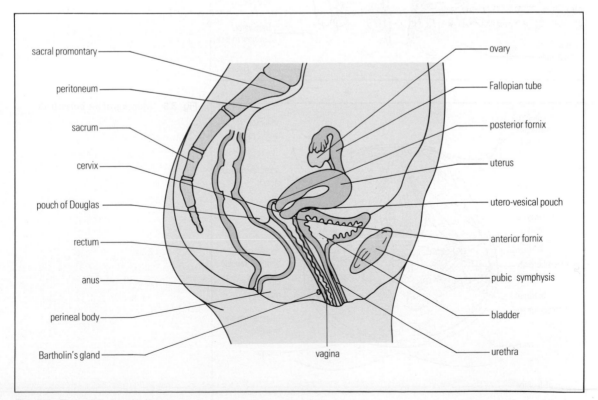

Fig. 3.1 The pelvis: lateral view.

Fig. 3.2 illustrates the distribution of pelvic muscles. The ischiorectal fossae lie lateral to the levator ani muscles, medial to the obturator internus muscles, and deep to the transverse perineal muscles. There is no barrier between this area and the retroperitoneal space higher up in the pelvis. As a result infection or bleeding into the fossae can spread very rapidly into the pelvis.

The pudendal vessels and nerves pass along the floor of the ischiorectal fossae. On each side, the internal pudendal artery runs through the fossa and divides into inferior haemorrhoidal, transverse perineal and perineal arteries, and also sends off small branches to the muscles. The internal pudendal nerve, arising from the second, third and fourth sacral nerves, passes through

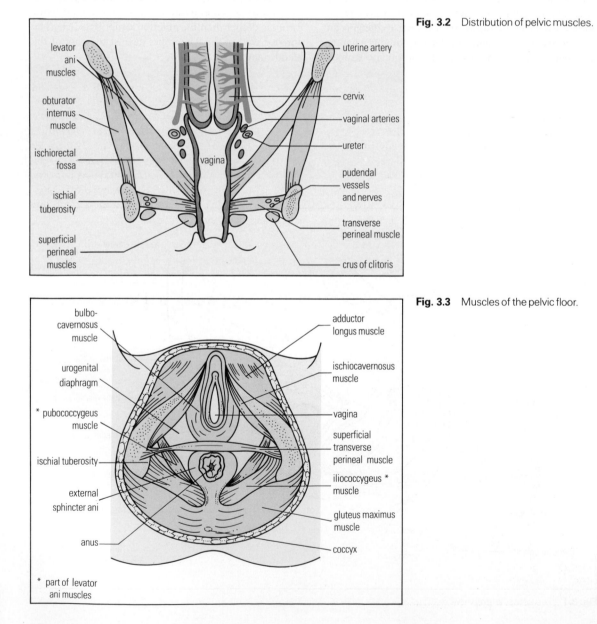

Fig. 3.2 Distribution of pelvic muscles.

Fig. 3.3 Muscles of the pelvic floor.

this region, dividing into numerous branches to supply structures in the area.

The muscles of the pelvic floor consist of the levator ani muscles, which lie at a deep level and other perineal muscles, which lie more superficially (Fig. 3.3).

The levator ani muscles arise on each side of the pelvis (from a line which passes backwards from the posterior surface of the pubic ramus) and pass over the internal surface of the obturator internus muscle to the ischial spine. From this origin, fibres on each side sweep downwards and backwards, interdigitating with each other in the midline around the upper portion of the vagina, bladder neck and rectum, and insert posteriorly into the lower portion of the sacrum and the coccyx. The levator ani muscles are bowl-shaped and form the pelvic diaphragm. Reflexes which raise the intra-abdominal pressure, such as coughing and sneezing will relax these muscles.

External to the levator ani muscles are the deep and superficial perineal muscles which provide support for structures in the lower pelvis. These consist of the bulbocavernosus muscles, the ischiocavernosus muscles, the superficial and deep transverse perineal muscles and the external anal sphincter.

The ischiocavernosus and bulbocavernosus muscles pass into the base of the clitoris. The superficial and deep perineal muscles extend from the sides of the pelvis and support the perineal body. They can be involved in tears and episiotomies at delivery.

The central point of the perineum is the perineal body. This is a musculo-fibrous structure, situated at a deep level between the vagina and the rectum. It acts as a keystone, with the transverse perineal muscles, bulbocavernosus muscles and the anal sphincter inserting into it. It may be damaged during obstetrical tears. The anal sphincter is under voluntary control. Its contraction adds to the capacity to close the exit of the anus and prevent the passage of flatus or faeces.

Blood supply

The blood supply to the uterus and vagina is provided mainly by the anterior branch of the internal iliac artery, from which the uterine, vaginal and obturator arteries arise (Fig. 3.4). The uterus receives its blood supply from the uterine arteries, which extend from the side walls of the pelvis and divide at the upper part of the cervix. The upper branches pass upwards, often dividing into two branches, to supply the body of the uterus. The lower branch divides into a series of small vessels extending downwards alongside the vagina.

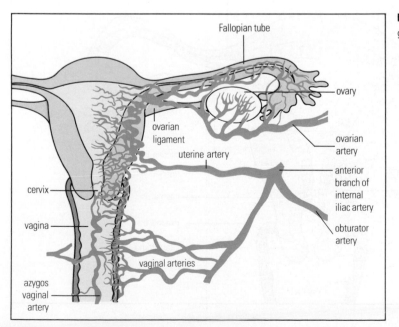

Fig. 3.4 Blood supply to the female genital tract.

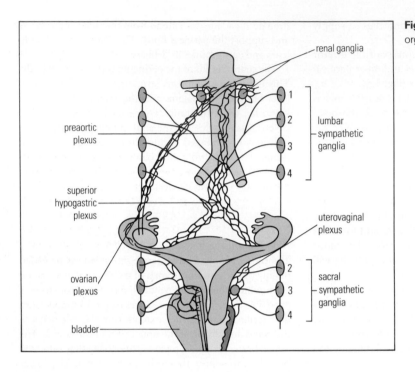

Fig. 3.5 Nerve supply to the pelvic organs.

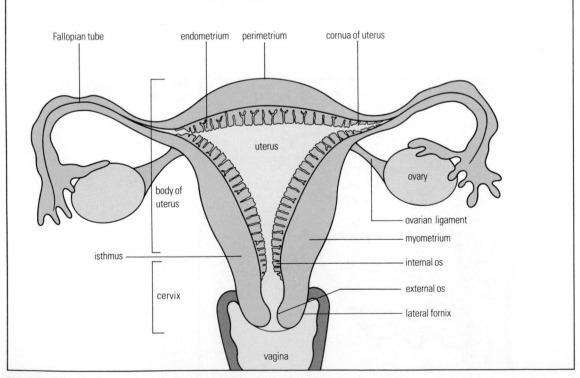

Fig. 3.6 The uterus.

The ovaries obtain blood from the ovarian arteries. These arise from the aorta on the posterior abdominal wall and run down behind the peritoneum. They pass in a fold of peritoneum from the back wall of the pelvis, over the pelvic brim towards each ovary; major terminal branches supply each Fallopian tube and anastamose with the uterine arteries on the underside of the tube.

Nerve supply

The pelvic organs are supplied by sympathetic and parasympathetic nerve plexuses. The sympathetic nerves arise from lumbar sympathetic ganglia, one, two, three and four. They pass from the preaortic plexus down to the uterovaginal plexus and ovary. The uterovaginal plexus rests in loose areolar tissue at the side of the cervix, at the level of the uterosacral folds of peritoneum. Parasympathetic fibres come from the second, third and fourth sacral nerves, and supply the pelvis through the uterovaginal plexus (Fig. 3.5).

Sympathetic nerve impulses relax the uterine muscle, especially during pregnancy. This effect is of pharma-

cological rather than physiological importance. Sensory impulses are also carried in the sympathetic nerves, and surgical division of these nerves may relieve pain in the pelvis.

The uterus

The uterus is a pear-shaped organ, divided into the body and cervix; a thin segment, the isthmus, lies between them (Fig. 3.6). During late pregnancy and labour, the isthmus is greatly expanded to form the lower uterine segment.

The uterine musculature is arranged in three ill-defined layers: an outer layer of longitudinal muscle, which passes anteriorly from the front of the isthmus, over the fundus of the uterus and down to the cervix; a thick layer of spiral myometrial fibres which encircles the cavity; and an inner layer of poorly defined circular muscle surrounding the ostia of the Fallopian tubes and the internal and external os of the cervix (Fig. 3.7). The uterus normally lies in anteversion and anteflexion and

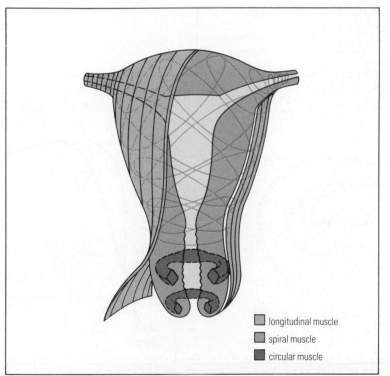

Fig. 3.7 Arrangement of the uterine musculature. (Courtesy of Gower Medical Publishing.)

☐ longitudinal muscle

☐ spiral muscle

■ circular muscle

is held in place by muscular and fibrous supports. The important muscular supports are the levator ani muscles, and wrapped around the pelvic organs, above the levator ani, is the pelvic fascia, which is firmly condensed in certain areas to produce fascial supports (Fig. 3.8). These are:

(i) Laterally, the transverse cervical ligaments, which pass from the lateral pelvic wall to the cervix near the internal os and which contain, in addition to

compressed fibrous tissue, the uterine vessels. In an upright position the ligaments suspend the uterus in a sling.

(ii) Posteriorly, the uterosacral ligaments, which are thinner and less effective as a support. They pass from the back of the cervix and fornices of the vagina to the anterior surface of the sacrum.

(iii) Anteriorly, the round ligaments, which stretch from the top of the uterus just in front of the

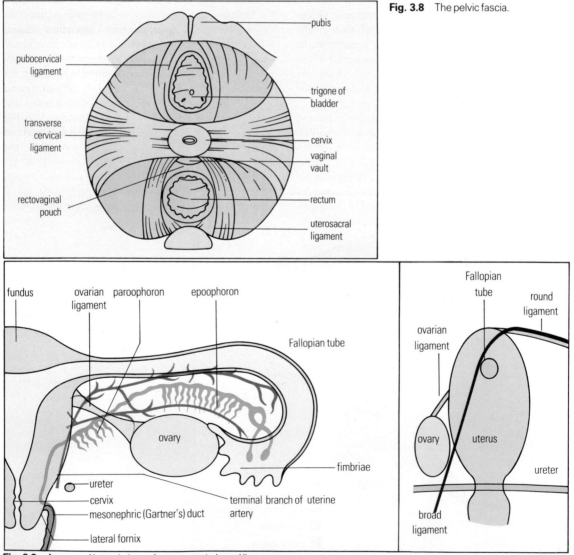

Fig. 3.8   The pelvic fascia.

Fig. 3.9   A rear and lateral view of structures in broad ligament.

cornua, along the path of the gubernaculum, around the side of the pelvis, under the peritoneum, enter the inguinal canal and terminate by becoming attached to the labium majora; they offer no major support and merely helps to hold the uterine fundus in anteversion. The broad ligament, although referred to as a ligament, has no major support function (Fig. 3.9).

The size of the uterine body in relation to the cervix changes at different times during a woman's life. At birth the uterine body is comparatively large, due to stimulation by oestrogens from the placenta, and is equal in length to the cervix, the ratio of body to cervix being 1:1. After birth, the placental source of oestrogen is no longer available and the uterine body shrinks, the cervix remaining relatively longer, with a body to cervix ratio of 1:2. At puberty, the uterine body is stimulated to grow, reversing this ratio (Fig. 3.10).

The vagina

The vagina is a fibromuscular elastic canal which starts as an opening in the external genitalia posterior to the urethra and anterior to the rectum. It extends from the hymen to the cervix of the uterus. Since the cervix extends in the anterior aspect of the superior end of the vagina the anterior wall is shorter than the posterior (8cm compared with 9–10cm respectively). The clefts produced by the cervix, projecting into the vagina are called fornices, an anterior and a posterior and two lateral fornices. The posterosuperior part of the vagina is covered by peritoneum whilst the anterior wall has no contact with it.

The important relations of the vagina are (see Figs 3.1 and 3.2):
- Anterior: bladder and urethra;
- Posterior: the perineal body, rectum and rectovaginal septum (Pouch of Douglas) which contains the small intestine, and,
- Laterally: the broad ligaments, ureters, uterine vessels, pelvic surface of the levator ani muscle, sphincter–urethra muscle, the greater vestibular glands (Bartholin's glands) and perineal muscles.

Thus any structure in the inferior part of the pelvic cavity can be palpated through the vagina particularly if bimanual palpation is used (see Fig. 3.18). Structures contained in the broad ligaments can be felt and when the ovary is enlarged from any pathological condition it can be examined from the vagina as well. The cervix of the uterus is of course palpable and it is also visible if the vagina is dilated with a speculum. The walls of the vagina are normally in contact with each other except where the cervix intervenes. They are made up of smooth muscle and lined with squamous epithelium.

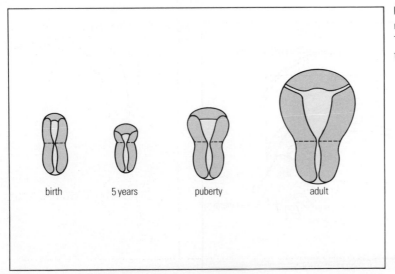

Fig. 3.10 The length of the cervix in relation to the length of the uterine body. The ratio of one to the other changes as the genital tract matures.

birth   5 years   puberty   adult

The ovaries and Fallopian tubes

The two ovaries are mainly solid ovoid structures about 3.5cm in length and 1.5–2.5cm thick. They are attached to the back of the broad ligament by the mesovarium on either side of the uterus and each is suspended from the cornua of the uterus by an ovarian ligament. The ovary is the only organ in the abdominal cavity which is not covered by the peritoneum. A part of the ovary, the hilum, is attached to the mesovarium and all nerves and vessels enter and leave at this point.

The relations of the ovary are similar to those of the Fallopian tube. The exact position of the ovary and tube vary considerably, sometimes near the pelvic brim and at other times in the uterorectal pouch. There are changes with age and parity; in infancy and childhood the ovary is a tiny and elongated structure with a smooth surface situated near the pelvic brim. After the menopause the ovary becomes small in size and shrivelled in appearance. The Fallopian tubes (uterine tubes) are approximately 10cm in length, they extend from the ovaries to the cornua of the uterus, one on either side. The lumen communicates with the uterine cavity at its inner end and the peritoneal cavity via its outer end and provides a potentially open canal from the vagina to the abdominal cavity. The Fallopian tube is divided into four parts (Fig. 3.11); the interstitial or intermural part, which is only 1–2cm in length and is the part which traverses the uterine wall approximately 1mm in diameter; the isthmus is the straight and narrow portion adjacent to the uterus and measures 2–3cm. Its walls are thick although the lumen is only 1–2mm in diameter. The ampulla is the wider thin-walled and tortuous outer portion approximately 5cm in length which leads to the infundibulum. The infundibulum is the trumpet-shaped outer end of the Fallopian tube with an opening into the peritoneal cavity, the abdominal ostia. The ostium is surrounded by fimbria, one of which is longer than the others and is directed towards the ovary. The fimbriated end is free of the broad ligament and curls back on itself so that the fimbria aim to embrace the ovary like tentacles of an octopus; this is important for fertility.

The bladder

The bladder is a hollow muscular organ, lying extra-peritoneally in the anterior part of the pelvis (see Fig. 3.1). The size and shape of the bladder vary with the amount of urine contained, but usually takes the form of an inverted pyramid, with the apex behind the pubic symphysis and the base against the wall of the peritoneal cavity.

The ureters enter the bladder at the posterolateral angles of the base, and the urethra leaves it inferiorly. The uterovesical pouch is formed by a reflection of the peritoneum covering the uterus and the superior surface of the bladder. The arterial blood supply is provided by the inferior and superior vesical branches of the internal iliac artery. The sympathetic nerve supply arises from

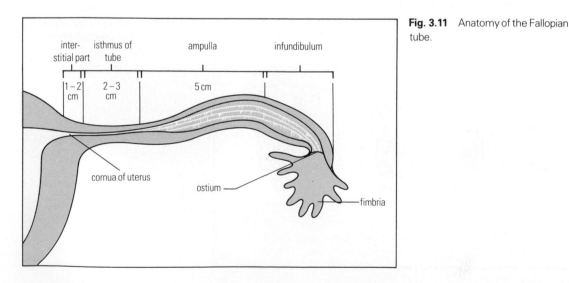

Fig. 3.11 Anatomy of the Fallopian tube.

the first and second lumbar segments, and the para-sympathetic fibres from sacral segments two, three and four (see Fig. 3.5).

The rectum

The rectum is a hollow tube approximately 12cm long, which joins the sigmoid colon to the anal canal (see Fig. 3.1). The lower third is embedded in pelvic fascia, the middle third is covered anteriorly by the peritoneum and the upper third is covered anteriorly and laterally by the peritoneum. There is no mesentery, the posterior border being retroperitoneal at all levels.

Posterior to the rectum lie the superior rectal artery, the third, fourth and fifth sacral nerves, the sympathetic trunk, and the sacral artery (the terminal branch of the aorta). Blood is supplied from the rectal arteries (branches of the internal iliac artery) which anasta-mose with branches of the inferior mesenteric artery superiorly, and the pudendal artery inferiorly.

Lymphatic drainage of the pelvic organs

The lymph nodes are located around the external and internal iliac arteries and the aorta (Fig. 3.12). The lower abdominal wall and the bladder drain into the external iliac nodes. The cervix drains into the internal iliac and obturator nodes, as does the body of the uterus; the uterine fundus may drain with the ovary into the para-aortic nodes. The perineum drains into the inguinal and femoral nodes. The external and internal iliac lymphatic vessels pass to the common iliac nodes and from there on to those adjacent to the aorta. Bacteria and tumour cells can pass along the lymphatic system to, or through, the lymph nodes.

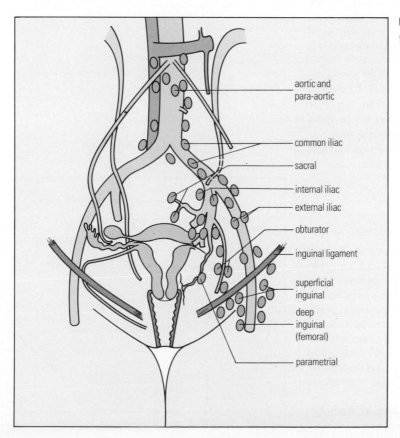

Fig. 3.12 Lymphatic drainage of the genital tract.

aortic and para-aortic

common iliac

sacral

internal iliac

external iliac

obturator

inguinal ligament

superficial inguinal

deep inguinal (femoral)

parametrial

The vulva

The vulva extends forwards from the anus to the hair covered pad of fat overlying the symphysis called the mons pubis. The lateral borders are the creases of the groins. The structures of the vulva are illustrated in Fig. 3.13 and consist of:

(i) An outer triangle with the sides formed of two hair covered 'lips' called the *labia majora* and the base formed by the perineum.

(ii) An inner triangle, the sides of which are the thinner *labia minora*, with a thin fold of skin, the *fourchette*, which joins the posterior ends, forming the base. Where the labia minora meets the apex of this inner triangle they split to enclose the small tip of the *clitoris*. The clitoris has a body and two crura, one on each side and is surrounded by erectile tissue.

(iii) The space inside the inner triangle, the *vestibule*, contains two orifices – anteriorly the smaller external urethral orifice and behind this the *introitus* to the vagina. The introitus is usually closed, unless gaping from obstetrical trauma or when air enters after separation of the labia minora. The introitus is partially covered by a thin membrane, the hymen, which may be stretched by the use of vaginal tampons, or by vaginal examination and is usually torn at first intercourse.

On each side, under cover of the posterior part of the labia minora, lies an oval pea-sized gland, Bartholin's gland which secretes clear lubricating fluid, especially during sexual excitement, through a duct which opens on each side at the posterior margin of the introitus. Infection or blockage of the duct or gland may lead to a Bartholin's abscess or Bartholin's cyst.

GYNAECOLOGICAL HISTORY

The taking of a history marks the beginning of a doctor–patient relationship at which time the doctor's attitude and sensitivity to the patient can be significant. The history should be taken in as relaxed and private setting as possible and the patient remain fully clothed at the first visit. The preliminary part of the interview should be devoted to putting the patient at ease and the questions and topics be of a very general nature. The doctor should observe the patient's general demeanour and emotional state from her facial expression, appearance and posture.

It is important when taking a history to remember that some patients find it embarrassing to discuss their gynaecological symptoms and that all questions should be asked in a professional, tactful manner. You should always allow the patient to relate the problem in her own words, because as she gains confidence she will disclose more significant and relevant information. Having obtained the broad outline in this way, specific details can be clarified by tactfully posed direct questions. One should not make assumptions about a patient's background e.g. that all women in the reproductive age group are both sexually active and heterosexual, for either or both may be incorrect.

A comprehensive and well taken history is of little use to the doctor or anyone else if it is not recorded in a legible and complete format. Good records should be accurate, objective, dated and signed. Pre-printed history forms or sheets are available in most hospitals and used to record basic information (Fig. 3.14). At the end of taking a history, it is good practice to ask the patient if she has any further questions or information she would like to add since some patients wait until they feel totally comfortable with the doctor before they give certain facts.

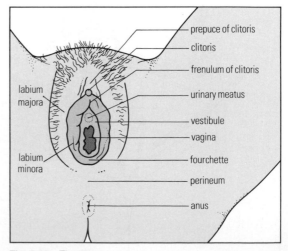

Fig. 3.13 The vulva.

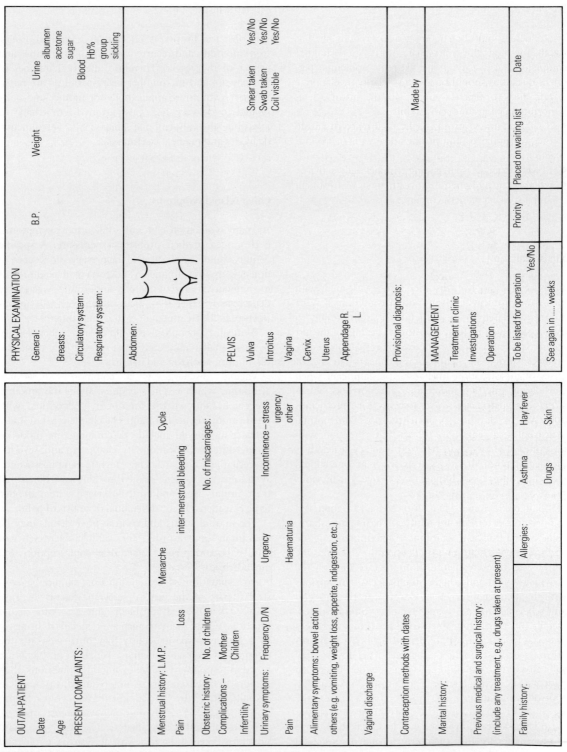

Fig. 3.14 Standard form.

Present complaint(s)

The patient should be encouraged to say why she has sought help at this particular time. After she has completed the history of her current problem(s) pertinent questions should be asked to clarify or elaborate certain facts or specific points in the history. It is important in all instances to establish:

- if she has a new problem, the recurrence of an old one, or similar to, but not identical with, a previous situation.
- to what extent it is interfering with her daily activity
- whether she had previous investigations or treatment and if so what were the results.

Menstrual history

Many gynaecological disorders are associated with menstrual problems and since other conditions may be indirectly related to menstruation, it is important to obtain a detailed menstrual history. The date of the last menstrual period is important (even if very approximate in the case of post-menopausal women). The age of onset of menstruation (menarche) is significant when considering infertility, secondary amenorrhoea, menstrual irregularities in adolescents or precocious puberty. The duration of menstrual loss and normal menstrual cycle length are recorded as a fraction, with the duration of loss as the numerator and cycle length as the denominator. If the cycle is irregular one should record the shortest and longest cycles over the previous year.

If pain is experienced in relation to menstruation, it is important to determine the nature of the pain (i.e. sharp, collicky or a dull ache, constant or intermittent), its site and radiation. The timing of its onset in relation to the period (i.e. the day before, hours before or with the flow) is relevant and whether the pain eases or worsens with the menstrual flow. The duration of the pain and any relieving or exacerbating factors should be noted. Details of the actual menstrual loss may be very important, particularly if the periods are heavy or if clots are passed. Assessment of the menstrual loss is very subjective and, therefore, varies widely between patients. In general, if the menstrual loss can be controlled by tampons it is not excessive, whereas the use of more than two packets of sanitary towels per period is taken to indicate a heavy loss, as is the passage of clots. The presence of intermenstrual or postcoital bleeding is highly significant.

Obstetric history

The obstetric history is relevant in several disorders, from infertility and recurrent abortion, to prolapse and cancer of the cervix. Therefore, the total number of pregnancies and the number of miscarriages are noted together with any complications for mother and baby related to delivery (e.g. postpartum haemorrhage or infection, thromboembolic phenomena, instrumental deliveries and perineal lacerations).

Other related symptoms

As many women present with some urinary symptoms, a clear idea of their problem is necessary. A specific enquiry should be made as to the presence or absence of urgency, dysuria, frequency, nocturia or haematuria. If incontinence is present it is very important to accurately determine whether it is stress, urgency or true incontinence, as the treatment of each is quite different.

Alimentary symptoms should be remembered since ovarian malignancy may first present as epigastric discomfort, anorexia and nausea.

Vaginal discharge is a common troublesome symptom, which requires enquiry about the amount, the colour and whether or not it is associated with micturition, soreness or pain. The characteristics of any pelvic pain should include determining the mode of onset, duration, location, its character, and severity, exacerbating and relieving factors and associated symptoms. Disorders related to the gastrointestinal tract, urinary tract and musculoskeletal system all have to be considered in the differential diagnosis of pain.

The marital status and contraceptive details may be relevant in some disorders, for example, the presence of an IUCD and menorrhagia, oral contraception and amenorrhoea.

An evaluation of sexual function should be considered part of the general screening history because many gynaecological problems interact with sexual function. Whilst many women are reluctant to bring up their problems spontaneously they often welcome the opportunity to discuss them if asked. If no problems are noted in response to the following three questions, then a more detailed enquiry is not required. (a) Are you sexually active? (b) Are you satisfied with your relationship? and (c) Do you have any pain with intercourse?

It is essential that a detailed medical history, past and present is taken and a review of all systems, family and personal history of social and occupational activities.

A general outline for a gynaecological and general history is given in Fig. 3.15.

Breast complaints

Bilateral breast tenderness that occurs regularly in the premenstrual phase in a spontaneously ovulating woman of reproductive age is not ordinarily a cause of concern. If the onset is recent and reflects a change from the usual pattern it requires evaluation. The report of a lump in the breast requires immediate assessment. Galactorrhoea can be a sign of an elevated prolactin level, but it can reflect chronic breast stimulation.

After completing the history the doctor should have formed some opinion as to the possible cause(s) of the problem(s) and this will point him/her to those areas that the history suggests are possibly the foci of dysfunction or pathology.

The examination of a gynaecological patient

A complete physical examination should be performed on all patients seen for the first time, regardless of the possible diagnosis. The general examination begins with observing the vital signs, followed by a careful general inspection. The examination should then proceed from head to toe. Particular emphasis should be placed on examination of the breasts, abdomen and pelvis. The pelvic and rectal examinations being carried out after the general physical examination has been completed.

IMPORTANT ASPECTS OF HISTORY TAKING	
1 details of principal complaint	4 family history
2 history of gynaecological problems	5 occupation and social history
menstruation – menarche, LMP and previous MP menstrual pattern obstetric history	6 allergies
vaginal and pelvic infection gynaecological operations urological history	7 medications, smoking, alcohol, drugs
pelvic pain vaginal bleeding sexual activity contraceptive measures	8 review of all systems CNS, CVS, respiratory, gastro-intestinal, genito-urinary, neuro-vascular, musculo-skeletal
3 previous medical and surgical history or any health problem	9 psychiatric problems

Fig. 3.15 Important aspects of history taking.

The reason for a full clinical examination and urinalysis being performed routinely is the possibility of the patient having an early non-gynaecological disorder as well. It is not uncommon to detect hypertension, diabetes mellitus, and pathological conditions of the breast (Fig. 3.16) in the gynaecological clinic. The abdominal examination should be full and not limited to a search for lesions arising from the pelvis. The groins should be routinely examined for the presence of lymph nodes.

Pelvic examination

The external genitalia should be both inspected and palpated. Observation should be made of the hair pattern, labia minora and majora, clitoris, urethra and total skin area to determine if there are any developmental abnormalities or skin lesions, or evidence of hormonal abnormalities. The vulval area should be palpated if there are any obvious lesions present. The Bartholin's glands are not normally palpable if they are healthy. Speculae come in a variety of sizes, and an appropriate size should be selected for the individual patient. From the history it can be assessed how easy it will be to pass a speculum e.g. if the patient uses tampons, is sexually active, or has had cervical smears taken previously, The majority of gynaecologists commence with a speculum examination of the vagina and cervix. Specimens of any vaginal discharge can be taken for culture and a cervical smear taken for cytology. The presence of any local lesion or atrophic change should be noted.

For most problems the examination will be performed with the patient in the dorsal or left lateral position at the examiner's choice. For assessing a prolapse or patient with incontinence the left lateral position, using a Sims'speculum is essential (Fig. 3.17).

Bimanual examination

Next, the examiner should palpate the vagina, cervix, uterus, adnexa (ovaries and tubes) and Pouch of Douglas. It is acceptable to use lubrication after all cultures and a cervical smear have been obtained. The index and middle fingers of the right hand are used to examine the vagina (Fig. 3.18). In some patients with a narrow introitus, only a single finger can be comfortably used. The abdominal hand should be used to sweep the pelvic organs downward while the vaginal hand is simultaneously elevating them. Using this manoeuvre, one can determine the size, mobility, position and consistency of the uterus. The adnexa should be checked for the presence of normal ovaries. The Fallopian tubes in health will not be palpable. Any masses found should be described as to location, size, consistency, mobility, and degree of tenderness. Finally, the Pouch of Douglas and uterosacral ligaments should be assessed for masses or nodularity.

A rectovaginal examination is indicated in some cases for it often helps assessing abnormalities in the rectovaginal septum, Pouch of Douglas and adnexal masses. A rectal examination is required if there is any suggestion of malignancy or in the presence of abnormal bleeding.

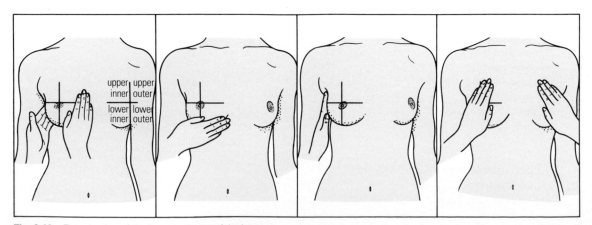

Fig. 3.16 Examination of the four quadrants of the breasts.

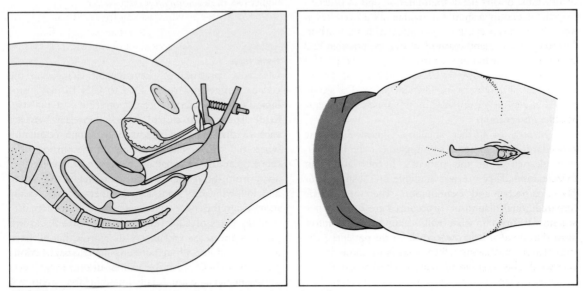

Fig. 3.17 Cuscoe's speculum inserted into the vagina so the cervix can be visualized (left). Examination in the lateral position with a Sims' speculum (right).

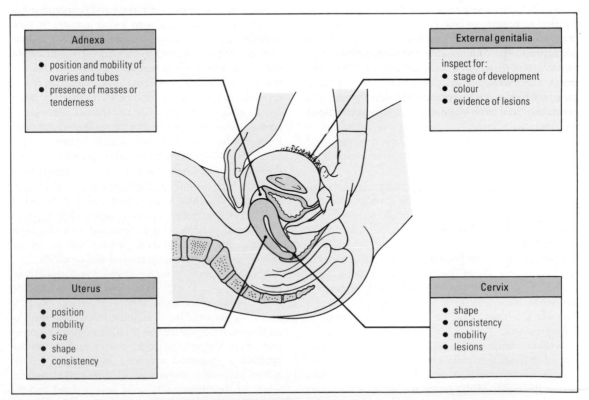

Adnexa

- position and mobility of ovaries and tubes
- presence of masses or tenderness

External genitalia

inspect for:
- stage of development
- colour
- evidence of lesions

Uterus

- position
- mobility
- size
- shape
- consistency

Cervix

- shape
- consistency
- mobility
- lesions

Fig. 3.18 Information from inspection and bimanual examination.

It must be remembered that many women are not comfortable during pelvic examination and in order to help the patient one should (i) explain all procedures in advance, (ii) keep eye to eye contact with the patient, (iii) keep the patient covered as far as possible and (iv) explain all the findings clearly.

Further observations

The purpose of further ancillary clinical diagnostic procedures is to compare or supplement the information gleaned from the patient's history and your examination. They are not infallible or substitutes for poor reasoning and examination. Therefore, before any additional diagnostic procedures are ordered one should ask oneself 'what will I gain from this information and will it help me to care for the patient?'. The purpose of establishing a diagnosis is to allow proper decisions to be made about treatment and prognosis.

SCREENING

Cervical Screening

Squamous cell carcinoma of the cervix arises from a non invasive precursor form, cervical intraepithelial neoplasia (CIN). Detection and destruction of the precursor state is therefore vital to prevent the development of a potentially fatal invasive cancer. Cytology screening of the superficial layers of the cervical epithelium is effective in picking up CIN and when widely used significantly reduces the morbidity and mortality of cervical squamous cell carcinoma.

In unscreened populations the prevalence of CIN is in the range of 6–7/1000 women. By contrast, the incidence of new disease in an already screened, and presumably disease-free population, is estimated at about 1/1000.

Epidemiological studies have estimated that the progression from CIN to invasive cancer takes a mean period of 10–15 years but the mean and the range is enormous. It is, for example, acknowledged that there is nowadays a more aggressive carcinoma tumour in young women.

Screening programs should be related to the relative risk of individual women rather than performed universally on an annual, 3 or 5 yearly basis. One must accept the reality of the world we live in and in most industrialized countries, sexual permissiveness is now

the rule. This pattern of behaviour puts women at a higher risk of developing cervical cancer.

Basic facts

CIN is a spectrum of premalignant changes in the cervical epithelium from CIN I to CIN III that histologically shows varying degrees of cellular atypia (Fig. 3.19). There is no clearly defined boundary between each of the atypia. The squamo-columunar junction where the atypias start is usually on the portio of the cervix near the external os. It may be found further away from the os during and after pregnancy, during and following oral contraceptive therapy and usually recedes into the endocervical canal after the menopause.

Many cases of CIN I (and possibly CIN II) do not progress and some spontaneously regress, but all have the potential for progression to malignancy. Lesions graded as CIN III are at the greatest risk for progression to malignancy and are usually found in larger abnormal transformation zones. However only about half of the proven cases of carcinoma in situ forms actually progress to invasive cancer.

The cause of cervical intraepithelial neoplasia is not known but is associated with sexual activity. Women with multiple sex partners are at an increased risk of CIN and males with multiple sex partners increase the risk of neoplasia for a female sex partner. Cigarette smoking is a contributory factor in increasing the risk of cervical neoplasia as is the commencement of intercourse at an early age. The non-barrier methods of contraception also appears to increase the risk for those women who have high risk sexual factors. Herpes simplex virus type II infection was suspected to increase the risk of cervical neoplasia but a definite causative role has not been identified. Papilloma virus infection is associated with an increased risk of CIN. Types 6 and 11 are associated with benign condylomata, whilst types 16 and 18 and possibly 31 are associated with neoplastic changes. Immunosuppressed patients are at an increased risk of developing intraepithelial neoplasia.

The false negative rate for properly performed cytology smears is 5–10%. The colposcope is used to evaluate the cervix if an abnormal cervical smear is present or persists. Usually multiple biopsy specimens of an abnormal transformation zone are needed for proper evaluation. Colposcopy and cytology findings do not establish a diagnosis and so a biopsy is necessary. Before outpatient therapy of CIN is carried out the whole of the abnormality must be visualized and the evaluation should be adequately able to exclude the presence of invasive carcinoma. The goal of treatment of intraepithelial neoplasia is eradication of all abnormal tissues using one form of ablation technique e.g. laser.

Follow up of patients treated for CIN consists of regular follow up cytology and, when appropriate, colposcopy.

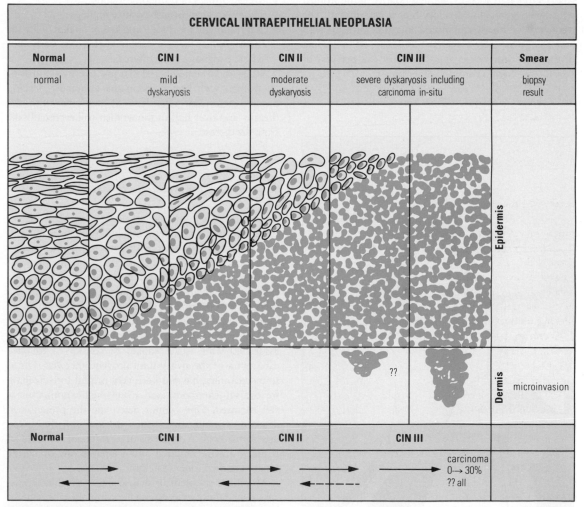

Fig.3.19 Diagrammatic representation of the precursors of cervical carcinoma CIN I, II and III which correspond to the former mild, moderate, severe and carcinoma in-situ. They are characterized by a progressive increase in the number of undifferentiated cells and a decrease in the differentiation of the superficial cells which parallel the increasing severity of the intraepithelial neoplasia. It is not known whether there is spontaneous regression of the abnormality from CIN III or what proportion of untreated lesions would become overt carcinoma.

Whilst microinvasion can develop from CIN III it is uncertain whether it develops directly from the other grades.

Breast screening

Unlike the situation with cervical cancer breast screening is not strictly a preventive measure, but an early detection exercise (Fig. 3.20). Its aim is to reduce mortality by detecting disease after the invasive state has occurred but still at an early stage. The inability to detect precancerous lesions limits the effectiveness of mammographic screening, although the potential reduction in mortality is substantial. About 1:10 to 1:14 women develop carcinoma of the breast during their lifetime. Risk factors only identify about a quarter of the women who will eventually develop breast carcinoma. The frequency of breast carcinoma increases directly with increasing age. Once a woman has developed carcinoma of the breast the risk is approximately 1% per year of developing carcinoma of the other breast.

There is evidence to suggest that screening women over 50 using mammography alone leads to a reduction in mortality from breast cancer by 35–40%. High standards and strict quality control are necessary to achieve these results. It is not a cheap test and needs to be set against the benefits of reduced mortality and improved prognosis for *some* women whose lesion is detected with early screening. Less radical treatment to cure some patients with early disease is also a benefit. Against the benefits has to be the potential and real cost of screening symptomless women which include:

- over treatment of borderline lesions
- anxiety created by false positive findings
- and the longer morbidity and loss of quality of life for those women whose lesion is detected early but whose prognosis is not altered.

It has to be remembered that just over two thirds of all women with breast carcinoma eventually develop distant metastases regardless of the type of initial therapy and over half of the women will eventually die from the disease.

Screening for other gynaecological cancers

At the present time the screening for other gynaecological cancers requires a high index of suspicion and investigation of women with symptoms. All women with post-menopausal or irregular pre-menopausal bleeding are candidates for a fractional curettage to exclude endometrial carcinoma. A biopsy should be carried out on any vulval lesion, no matter where its location or the patient's age to exclude vulval carcinoma.

Any woman with a pelvic mass particularly if it is associated with ascites should be considered to have carcinoma of the ovary until proven otherwise. Ultrasound scanning has not been very helpful for screening for ovarian carcinoma and a bimanual examination is still required. One cannot determine the presence or absence of malignant ovarian disease with the naked eye. A histological diagnosis of a reasonable amount of tissue is always required and a laparoscopy or needle biopsy are therefore not helpful.

The main problem in diagnosing trophoblastic disease is the failure to recognise the symptoms and signs of hydatidiform mole. Ultrasound has made the diagnosis easier and beta HCG is an excellent tumour marker.

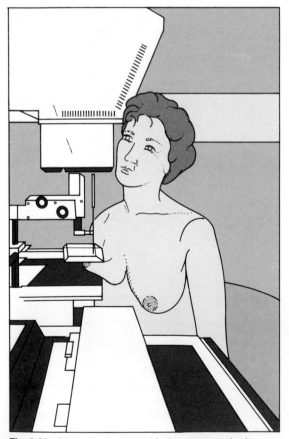

Fig. 3.20 Mammography used for breast screening in women aged 50 and over, in particular.

4   Gynaecological Symptoms

INTRODUCTION

All patients present with a symptom or symptoms and it is from the history given with appropriate direct questioning that possible causes for the symptoms can be considered. Whilst there is an inevitable overlap with gynaecological conditions every effort has been made to discuss the individual symptoms on their own merits. Appropriate cross reference to conditions and symptoms are made throughout.

AMENORRHOEA

Amenorrhoea is the absence of menstrual discharge from the uterus. This can be physiological at three stages in a women's life: before puberty, during pregnancy and lactation and after the menopause (Fig. 4.1). Other than at these times amenorrhoea is a symptom indicating the presence of an anatomic, genetic, biochemical, physiological or emotional abnormality. The pathophysiology of amenorrhoea should be considered in relation to the physiology of menstruation. A series of interrelated factors are required for the visible discharge of menstrual blood (see Figs 2.15 and 2.16).

(i) an endometrium responsive to hormonal stimulation;
(ii) an intact hypothalamic/pituitary ovarian axis, where secretion of GnRH stimulates the pituitary to release FSH and LH;
(iii) secretion of oestrogen from the ovary and after ovulation the additional secretion of progesterone as a result of FSH and LH stimulation;
(iv) patency and continuity of the uterus, cervix, vagina and vaginal orifice.

A defect in any one or more of these may result in amenorrhoea.

It is usual to classify amenorrhoea as either primary, i.e. the girl who has never menstruated, or secondary, when she has previously menstruated. Amenorrhoea may be suspected as being pathological in a girl aged 14 when she shows no indication of menstruation and secondary characteristics, or in any girl aged 16 regardless of whether or not there are secondary sexual characteristics. It should also be investigated when there

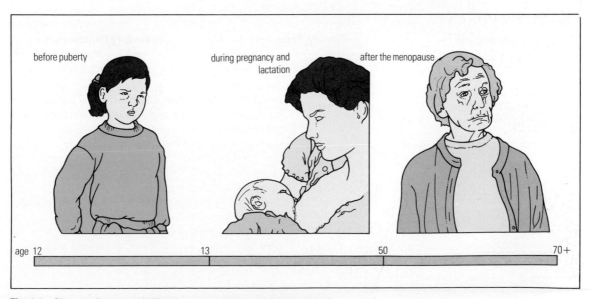

before puberty   during pregnancy and lactation   after the menopause

age 12   13   50   70+

Fig. 4.1   Phases of a woman's life where amenorrhoea is 'physiological'.

is cessation of periods in a woman, of any age, who previously had a normal menstrual cycle. It is not uncommon for a spontaneous menopause to occur in some women in the their mid-thirties and a significant number of teenagers have amenorrhoea lasting 2–12 months during the first two or three years following their menarche. Fig. 4.2 summarizes the main causes of amenorrhoea.

Cryptomenorrhoea

True amenorrhoea must be differentiated from crypto-menorrhoea, where the pituitary gland, ovaries and uterus are functioning normally, but there is an obstruction to the outflow of blood. This may simply be due to an imperforate hymen or another membrane found higher in the vagina. There may be an association with cyclical pain once ovulation occurs. Some of the menstrual blood is absorbed with each 'period' so that the

usual age of referral is between 13 and 16 years of age.

The treatment is simply to incise the membrane with two crossing incisions and allow the blood to drain spontaneously (Fig. 4.3). Any other treatment carries with it the danger of ascending infection and subsequent sterility.

Primary amenorrhoea

Some cases of amenorrhoea merely reflect a constitutional delay in the menarche, which may be familial. The average age for the menarche is between 11 and 13 years and it is not usually necessary to investigate primary amenorrhoea before 16 years.

Causes
Fig. 4.4 illustrates some of the possible causes of

AMENORRHOEA		
Physiological	**Primary Pathological**	**Secondary Pathological**
false amenorrhoea: cryptomenorrhoea	gonadal failure, absent or rudimentory uterus	surgical or radiotherapeutic ablation
true amenorrhoea: pre-puberty, pregnancy, lactation, menopause		endocrine disorders, malnutrition, obesity

Fig. 4.2 Major causes of amenorrhoea.

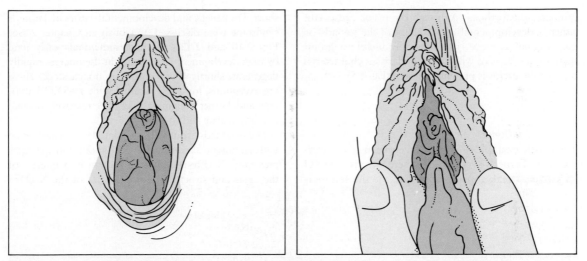

Fig. 4.3 Cryptomenorrhoea. Imperforate hymen with exposure of the collected menstrual blood and its release.

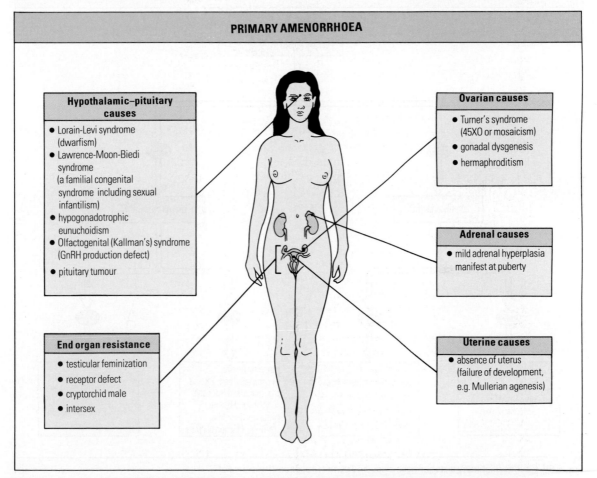

PRIMARY AMENORRHOEA

Hypothalamic–pituitary causes

- Lorain-Levi syndrome (dwarfism)
- Lawrence-Moon-Biedi syndrome (a familial congenital syndrome including sexual infantilism)
- hypogonadotrophic eunuchoidism
- Olfactogenital (Kallman's) syndrome (GnRH production defect)
- pituitary tumour

End organ resistance

- testicular feminization
- receptor defect
- cryptorchid male
- intersex

Ovarian causes

- Turner's syndrome (45XO or mosaicism)
- gonadal dysgenesis
- hermaphroditism

Adrenal causes

- mild adrenal hyperplasia manifest at puberty

Uterine causes

- absence of uterus (failure of development, e.g. Mullerian agenesis)

Fig. 4.4 Some causes of primary amenorrhoea.

GYNAECOLOGICAL SYMPTOMS

primary amenorrhoea. Although the major causes are either a developmental abnormality of the gonads or uterovaginal agenesis, it is clinically useful to group them on the basis of whether secondary sex characteristics and the uterus is present or absent (Fig. 4.5).

Turner's syndrome
The classic example of gonadal agenesis, usually referred to as Turner's syndrome is where there is a 45XO karyotype, streak gonads are present and the stature is

short. The genetic and developmental causes of Turner's syndrome were discussed previously in Chapter 2 (see Figs 2.10 and 2.11). In these individuals early fetal ovarian development is normal, but the oocytes rapidly degenerate shortly after the primary oocyte stage. There are exceptions, for a few women with a 45XO karyotype and Turner's stigmata may have relatively normal ovaries, ovulate and conceive.

Streak gonads are usually associated with a karyotype with an absent X chromosome in about half the cases presented, X chromosomal mosaicism in a quarter of the cases and structural abnormalities of the X chro-

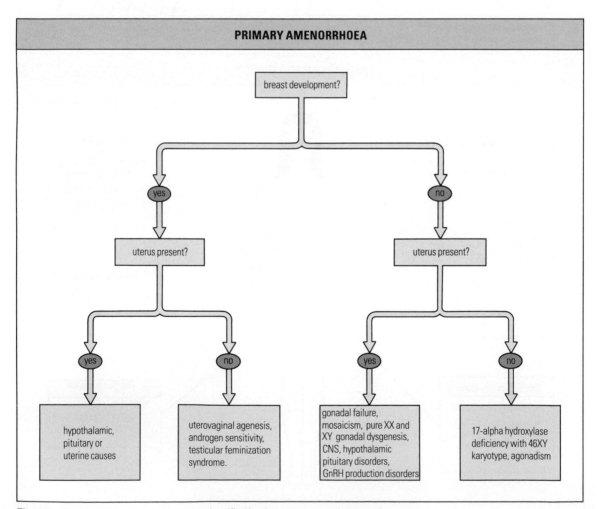

Fig. 4.5 Causes of primary amenorrhoea classified by the presence or absence of breast development and a uterus.

42

mosome in the remainder. After 45XO the most common abnormality is a 45XO/46XX mosaic. These individuals have few somatic abnormalities and breast development and a more normal stature is common. Although, if these women conceive there is higher frequency of gonadal dysgenesis in the offspring.

One third of the individuals with gonadal failure will have major cardiovascular or renal abnormalities. If there is gonadal failure and a Y chromosome present there is a risk of gonadal malignancy in later life. Mullerian agenesis (failure of fusion of the Mullerian ducts) comprises absence of the vagina and a total or partial absence of the uterus. It is also associated with renal and skeletal abnormalities. These conditions are discussed further in Chapter 6.

Investigations
A detailed history and general examination is necessary, making a particular note of the patient's height, weight, general characteristics, secondary sex characteristics and development. Some of the tests used to establish the cause of amenorrhoea are listed in Fig. 4.6.

TESTS USED TO IDENTIFY THE CAUSE OF AMENORRHOEA (OR OLIGOMENORRHOEA)	
Test	**Rationale**
Serum FSH and LH	to diagnose hypergonadotropic amenorrhoea; two or three measurements are often necessary; check for polycystic ovarian disease
Prolactin	to check for pituitary microadenoma or tumour
Serum TSH and thyroxine	to exclude thyroid dysfunction as a cause of amenorrhoea, screening for autoimmune thyroid disease
Serum testosterone, androstendione	to check for virilizing factor, polycystic ovarian syndrome
Serum cortisol (morning)	screening for adrenal insufficiency
Karotype	to test women with primary amenorrhoea, incomplete sexual maturation or gonadal dysgenesis
Serum oestradiol	to diagnose oestrogen deficiency
Ovarian biopsy	for evidence of follicles and a perifollicular lymphocytic infiltrate; choice of therapy rarely depends on results

Fig. 4.6 Tests used to identify the cause of amenorrhoea (or oligomenorrhoea). Often the history and physical examination may be sufficient to indicate a diagnosis, and so these tests should be used selectively.

If breast development is absent, then an FSH examination will identify hypergonadotrophic hypogonadism if it is low and gonadal dysgenesis if it is high. If normal this may reflect a delay in the onset of puberty. X-rays of the wrist joints allows assessment of any discrepancy between bone age and chronological age.

To diagnose pituitary microadenomas or tumours, the prolactin level and radiological assessment of the pituitary fossa are required (this is discussed further below). If the prolactin level is raised, thyroid function should also be assessed by TSH and thyroxine determinations. This may indicate thyroid dysfunction as a cause for the amenorrhoea. Other endocrine disturbances which cause amenorrhoea, such as adrenal insufficiency, can be assessed by the early morning serum cortisol level, although an ACTH stimulation test may be required to confirm this diagnosis.

If there is any evidence of virilization the serum testosterone and androstendrone levels should be assessed. An indication of polycystic ovarian disease (excessive androgen secretion) may be given by the LH:FSH ratio.

If a high FSH level suggests gonadal dysgenesis then the karyotype should be determined. If a Y chromosome is found the gonads will require removal at some time because of the risk of malignant change. The woman should not, however, be told about the Y chromosome, but merely told she has an abnormality of the autosomes which indicates malignancy might occur if the 'ovaries' are left *in-situ*. If a Y chromosome is absent then the precise state of the internal pelvic organs should be assessed by laparoscopy. Ultrasound of the abdomen and pelvis can confirm the presence (or absence) of the ovaries, uterus and kidneys, but is less helpful for determining maldevelopment.

Management of primary amenorrhoea

The treatment of primary amenorrhoea depends upon an accurate diagnosis of the underlying condition and then providing the appropriate therapy, if practical. Sexual maturation and menstruation can be induced when there is a uterus present either by gonadotrophin therapy or by inducing oestrogen withdrawal bleeding by giving hormone replacement therapy, e.g. the combined oestrogen and progesterone pill. If the ovaries are absent it is impossible for the woman to conceive.

In cases of cryptomenorrhoea the surgical procedures described above may be required to establish a patent exit from the uterus, although sometimes more complex operations are required to form the vagina.

Secondary amenorrhoea

Secondary amenorrhoea is due to an acquired lesion and thus the causes are different from those of primary amenorrhoea. Secondary amenorrhoea is said to be present following an absence of menstruation for a variable period of time, but at least three months and usually six months or longer. This definition therefore includes the physiological states of pregnancy and lactation, which are the commonest causes of secondary amenorrhoea. One should be aware of the occasional anomaly of the girl presenting with symptoms of secondary amenorrhoea who has, in fact, not had true menstruation, but merely hormone 'withdrawal bleeding'. Any acquired lesion of the individual links in the chain necessary for normal menstruation may cause secondary amenorrhoea.

Causes

The causes of secondary amenorrhoea are depicted in Fig. 4.7. Some of the pathological causes are associated with lack of secondary sexual characteristics (sexual infantilism), but in the majority sexual development is apparently normal, although there may be evidence of varying degrees of hirsutism or virilization.

Emotional or psychological disturbances can interfere with the normal pituitary/ovarian/uterine functions by virtue of a central cortical effect on hypothalamic action. A classic example of this is a medical student who came to the University from a rural community. She had menstruated normally during her schooldays, but was amenorrhoeic for five years until the first day of her Final MB examination. Thereafter her periods were regular and she subsequently conceived easily after marriage.

Organic conditions that also affect hypothalamic function include encephalitis, meningitis, trauma or tumours. Drugs, such as phenothiazines, digoxin, reserpine and ganglion blocking agents, may also affect the hypothalamus. The higher centres of the brain are also susceptible to marked weight changes, for example as with anorexia nervosa.

Pituitary tumours, particularly microadenomas, may cause amenorrhoea. These are associated with hyperprolactinaemia with or without galactorrhoea. A rarer condition nowadays is pituitary necrosis, Sheehan's syndrome, following post-partum haemorrhage and hypotensive shock in pregnancy or labour.

Ovarian function can be disturbed by surgery, radiation or it may cease prematurely. The possible causes of

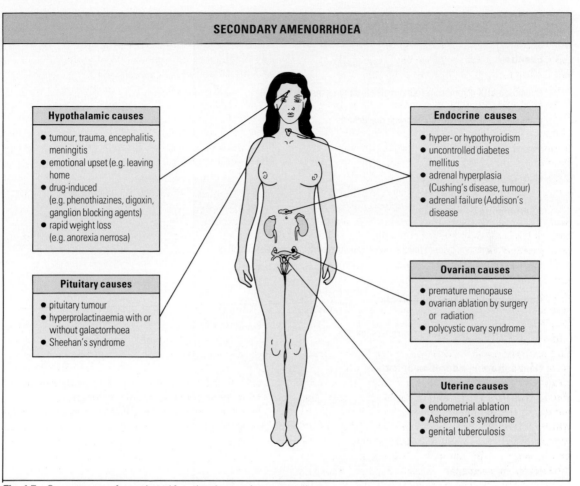

SECONDARY AMENORRHOEA

Hypothalamic causes
- tumour, trauma, encephalitis, meningitis
- emotional upset (e.g. leaving home)
- drug-induced (e.g. phenothiazines, digoxin, ganglion blocking agents)
- rapid weight loss (e.g. anorexia nerrosa)

Pituitary causes
- pituitary tumour
- hyperprolactinaemia with or without galactorrhoea
- Sheehan's syndrome

Endocrine causes
- hyper- or hypothyroidism
- uncontrolled diabetes mellitus
- adrenal hyperplasia (Cushing's disease, tumour)
- adrenal failure (Addison's disease)

Ovarian causes
- premature menopause
- ovarian ablation by surgery or radiation
- polycystic ovary syndrome

Uterine causes
- endometrial ablation
- Asherman's syndrome
- genital tuberculosis

Fig. 4.7 Some causes of organic and functional secondary amenorrhoea.

premature ovarian failure are given in Fig. 4.8. The polycystic ovary (Stein–Leventhal) syndrome in which there is an imbalance of hormone production from the ovary with an elevation of androgens causes secondary amenorrhoea. However, the typical history is usually that of infrequent periods, which are often heavy, obesity and hirsutism.

Uterine causes of amenorrhoea include removal of the endometrium or obliteration of the uterine cavity (Asherman's syndrome). The endocrine causes include hypo- or hyperthyroidism, uncontrolled diabetes, adrenal hyperplasia, disease or tumour and adrenal failure. Other causes of secondary amenorrhoea include the so-called general causes such as nutritional de-

ficiencies, strenuous physical activity, environmental changes etc. and these are usually related to one of the above.

Investigations
General
Thorough investigation is indicated to determine the cause of secondary amenorrhoea or oligomenorrhoea (infrequent periods) for they have a similar aetiology. The history gives important clues and indicates the appropriate special investigations which may be required or should be performed. These are essentially

45

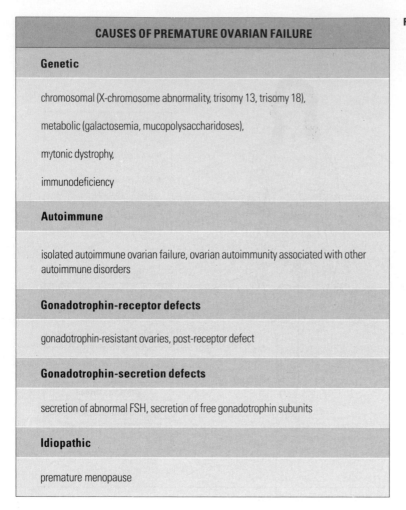

Fig. 4.8 Causes of ovarian failure.

CAUSES OF PREMATURE OVARIAN FAILURE
Genetic
chromosomal (X-chromosome abnormality, trisomy 13, trisomy 18),
metabolic (galactosemia, mucopolysaccharidoses),
mytonic dystrophy,
immunodeficiency
Autoimmune
isolated autoimmune ovarian failure, ovarian autoimmunity associated with other autoimmune disorders
Gonadotrophin-receptor defects
gonadotrophin-resistant ovaries, post-receptor defect
Gonadotrophin-secretion defects
secretion of abnormal FSH, secretion of free gonadotrophin subunits
Idiopathic
premature menopause

the same as mentioned in relation to primary amenorrhoea, excluding chromosomal analysis and accepting that the uterus is present and has been functioning and menstruation has occurred (see Fig. 4.6).

The history and examination may indicate emotional stress or psychological factors, weight loss, excessive or competitive exercise and the taking of drugs for whatever purpose. Fig. 4.9 shows a flow chart indicating one pattern of investigation starting with the exclusion of pregnancy. Apart from clinical examination this may require an ultrasound examination of the pelvis and/or the estimation of the beta HCG subunit for exclusion of pregnancy inside or outside the uterus. Indeed, the diagnostic possibilities suggested by history and clinical examination alone are considered in Figs 4.4 and 4.7.

If pregnancy is excluded it is reasonable to determine if there is chronic anovulation, uterine abnormalities, premature ovarian failure and dysfunction or failure in the pituitary gland or hypothalamus.

Prolactin levels
Prolactin is the hormone which is secreted by the anterior lobe of the pituitary gland to induce lactation. It suppresses the production of LH. An elevated prolactin level with or without galactorrhoea will indicate the necessity for excluding a pituitary microadenoma or tumour, before considering bromocriptine therapy to lower the prolactin level. Galactorrhoea as a symptom

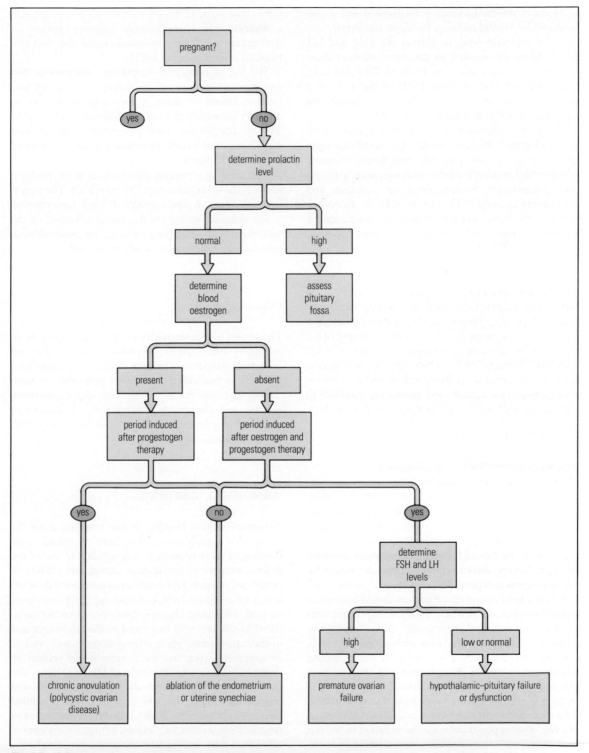

Fig. 4.9 A flow chart for considering the main groups of causes of secondary amenorrhoea or oligomenorrhoea.

is discussed later in the chapter. Prolactin release is also increased by thyroid releasing hormone and stress.

If the prolactin level is normal the FSH and LH levels should be assessed to determine whether there is pituitary dysfunction (low levels of FSH and LH), premature menopause (high FSH) or the polycystic ovarian (Stein–Leventhal) syndrome in which the LH:FSH ratio is greater than 3:1.

If the prolactin level is lower than normal, some gynaecologists will then measure the blood oestrogen level, but others will proceed immediately to assess whether the woman's uterus responds with a period after progestogen therapy alone, or oestrogen and progestogen together. This is in order to determine whether the basic problem is one of anovulation or abnormality of the endometrium if there is no response.

Surgical investigations
Surgical investigations include laparoscopy for inspection and possible biopsy of the ovaries (although a laparotomy may be preferable for a proper biopsy of the ovaries) or hysteroscopy to inspect the uterine cavity for synechia. A diagnostic curettage may be appropriate, if genital tuberculosis is suspected, in order to obtain endometrium for culture and guinea pig inoculation, although in the UK this condition is very rare nowadays.

Management of secondary amenorrhoea
Having established the cause for the secondary amenorrhoea the debate that remains is – is it appropriate or worthy of treatment? This usually depends on whether the woman wishes to become pregnant or not. Prolactin secretory tumours may be controlled by bromocriptine therapy (2.5 mg tds) and sometimes in conjunction with surgery. Non-prolactin secreting tumours should be excised if surgically possible.

Women with excessive weight loss should be advised to gain weight, although this is difficult in patients with anorexia nervosa and they should receive psychiatric treatment. Those women who embark on strenuous exercise and are highly competitive by nature should be advised to reduce these activities if they desire a pregnancy. Such women and those with polycystic ovarian syndrome often require induction of ovulation with clomiphene citrate in order to conceive. Because of the risk of unopposed oestrogen stimulation in women with polycystic ovarian syndrome producing endometrial hyperplasia and carcinoma, progestogen therapy

for the first 10 to 12 days of each month is appropriate.

Women with hypothalamic pituitary failure or dysfunction can have ovulation induced with gonadotrophins or intermittent LHRH.

The use of oestrogens to prevent osteoporosis and coronary artery disease in women with premature ovarian failure or those women with hypothalamic pituitary failure has also to be considered, but it must be used in conjunction with progestogens for at least 10–12 days per month. Hormone therapy is discussed further in Chapter 8.

One cause of secondary amenorrhoea not considered above is the so-called post-pill amenorrhoea. The reason is simply that it is now considered that if menstruation is not resumed within six months of cessation of the 'pill' there is an underlying cause for the amenorrhoea, namely one of the causes already mentioned.

Oligomenorrhoea

The causes of oligomenorrhoea are similar to those of secondary amenorrhoea. Several years of irregular and infrequent menses may precede secondary amenorrhoea and this is particularly true with premature ovarian failure. The majority of women with oligomenorrhoea ovulate and menstruate intermittently. Induction of ovulation may be required for these women if they wish to become pregnant.

ABNORMAL BLEEDING

Abnormal uterine bleeding is any bleeding from the uterus that significantly differs from menstrual cycle bleeding. This may occur at any age and is one of the most common gynaecological complaints. When it occurs around puberty or the menopausal periods of life it may be associated with endocrinological disturbances or with neoplastic changes. Disturbance of the menstrual loss is generally functional in the adolescent and in the reproductive era is related to pregnancy and its complications, but becoming increasingly related to organic disease in the later years of life (Fig. 4.10). The use of hormonal preparations for contraceptive and therapeutic purposes may be associated with abnormal bleeding and has to be distinguished from functional or organic disease. Organic lesions, benign or malignant, other than those arising from the uterus may also be the cause of abnormal bleeding.

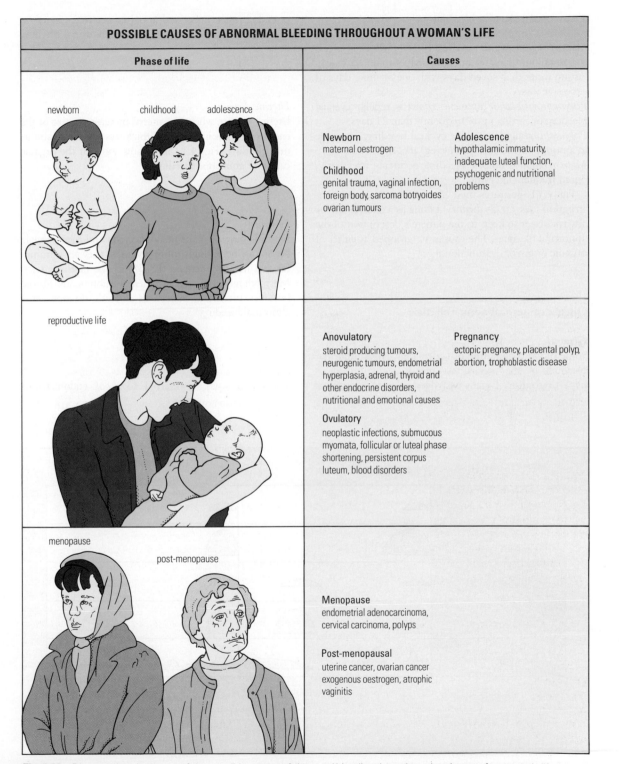

POSSIBLE CAUSES OF ABNORMAL BLEEDING THROUGHOUT A WOMAN'S LIFE

Phase of life	Causes
newborn childhood adolescence	**Newborn** maternal oestrogen **Childhood** genital trauma, vaginal infection, foreign body, sarcoma botryoides ovarian tumours **Adolescence** hypothalamic immaturity, inadequate luteal function, psychogenic and nutritional problems
reproductive life	**Anovulatory** steroid producing tumours, neurogenic tumours, endometrial hyperplasia, adrenal, thyroid and other endocrine disorders, nutritional and emotional causes **Ovulatory** neoplastic infections, submucous myomata, follicular or luteal phase shortening, persistent corpus luteum, blood disorders **Pregnancy** ectopic pregnancy, placental polyp, abortion, trophoblastic disease
menopause post-menopause	**Menopause** endometrial adenocarcinoma, cervical carcinoma, polyps **Post-menopausal** uterine cancer, ovarian cancer exogenous oestrogen, atrophic vaginitis

Fig. 4.10 Diagram showing some of the possible causes of abnormal bleeding throughout the phases of a woman's life.

49

Terms used to describe bleeding

Menorrhagia is regular cyclical bleeding which is excessive in amount (greater than normal) or in duration, e.g. lasting more than seven days with one or more days of excessive loss.

Polymenorrhoea or epimenorrhoea is regular cyclical bleeding occurring more frequently than 21 days.

Polymenorrhagia is regular cyclical bleeding, excessive in amount and also frequency, eg. 10/21.

Metrorrhagia is uterine bleeding occurring irregularly, but at frequent intervals.

Fig. 4.11 illustrates these abnormal patterns of menstruation. As far as history taking is concerned it is always better to keep to the patient's description of the abnormal bleeding. The causes are grouped as either of organic origin or dysfunctional.

Organic causes of abnormal bleeding

General
Some blood coagulation disorders may cause abnormal bleeding in the uterus, as may hypothyroidism or hyperthyroidism. Excess oestrogens, due to exogenous or endogenous causes and impaired oestrogen inactivation as with liver disease, will cause abnormal bleeding too.

Uterine disease
Uterine disease where the uterus increases in size or the endometrium is increased in thickness will cause abnormal bleeding. Fig. 4.12 illustrates some of the organic causes of abnormal bleeding.

Fibroids
Fibroids may produce heavy periods and menorrhagia becoming increasingly more profuse if they are intramural and thereby increase the size of the uterine cavity. Metrorrhagia may occur when a submucous fibroid becomes ulcerated. Subserous fibroids do not cause abnormal bleeding.

Adenomyosis
Adenomyosis is an internal form of endometriosis

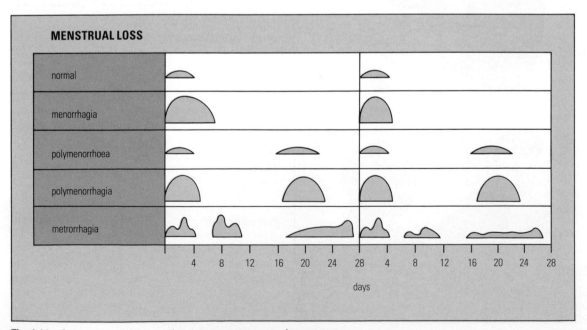

Fig. 4.11   Comparison of the normal and abnormal patterns of menstruation

which is associated with the uterine size being increased two to threefold. Characteristically it is associated with symptoms of menorrhagia, although sometimes polymenorrhoea. It is also associated with painful periods (dysmenorrhoea, see below).

Endometrial polyps
Endometrial polyps usually cause metrorrhagia.

Cervical polyps, erosions or carcinomas
These may cause irregular bleeding usually after contact, e.g. post-coital bleeding.

Uterine congestion
An ill-defined and doubtful entity sometimes called chronic subinovulation following pregnancy which is thought to be associated with menorrhagia.

Ovarian disease
Follicular cysts
Follicular cysts usually cause polymenorrhoea which may be related to high oestrogen levels produced by these cysts which fail to rupture.

Ovarian tumours
In general ovarian tumours, benign or malignant, do not cause bleeding. An exception are the oestrogen producing tumours e.g. granulosa cell tumours which in the reproductive years may give rise to heavy periods at irregular intervals.

Endometriosis
A 'chocolate cyst' may cause polymenorrhoea or polymenorrhagia by upsetting normal ovarian function, but the precise mechanism is unknown. Other symptoms are more likely to occur such as dysmenorrhoea or dyspareunia.

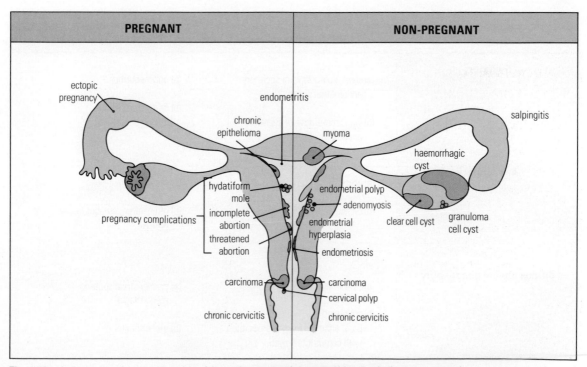

Fig. 4.12   A diagrammatic representation of the main causes of abnormal bleeding in the pregnant and non pregnant states.

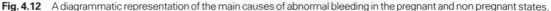

Tubal disease

Salpingo-oophoritis

Salpingo-oophoritis is inflammation of the Fallopian tubes and ovaries caused by bacterial infection. Whilst it may have no effect on the menstrual cycle chronic infection with recurrent subacute infection is associated with polymenorrhoea often proceeding to polymenorrhagia. This is a reflection of the involvement of the uterus in the inflammatory process.

Pregnancy

Irregular bleeding may occur as one of the complications of early pregnancy, e.g. decidual bleeding, ectopic pregnancy or trophoblastic disease (hydatidiform mole or choriocarcinoma) (Fig. 4.12). These are discussed further in Chapter 6, Gynaecological Conditions.

Dysfunctional uterine bleeding

Dysfunctional uterine bleeding is excessive bleeding without an identifiable organic cause, either genital or extragenital. It is one of the commonest gynaecological symptoms requiring investigation. It is most frequently due to abnormalities of endocrine origin affecting the synchronized activity of the pituitary/ovarian/uterine axis, and in particular menstrual cycles in which ovulation does not occur (anovulation). Fig. 4.13 summarizes the main features and symptoms of dysfunctional uterine bleeding.

Dysfunctional bleeding associated with ovulation

This is characterized by regular menstrual cycles of approximately the same duration. The patterns of bleeding include the following:

(i) *Midcycle spotting.* Scanty, bloody intermenstrual discharge due to decrease in oestrogen following ovulation at midcycle.

(ii) *Frequent periods.* Polymenorrhoea associated with a short pre-ovulatory follicular phase.

(iii) *Luteal phase deficiency.* This is associated with pre-menstrual spotting when the luteal phase is abruptly shortened as a result of corpus luteal

	POSSIBLE FEATURES	POSSIBLE SYMPTOMS
Ovulatory	(a) short proliferative or secretory endometrial phase (b) long proliferative or secretory endometrial phase	(a) polymenorrhoea (b) infrequent periods (oligomenorrhoea)
Anovulatory	(a) acyclical (b) cyclical	(a) metrorrhagia (b) often infrequent, but heavy, periods
Corpus luteum abnormality	(a) deficiency (b) prolonged (rare, although may be associated with corpus luteal cyst)	(a) premenstrual spotting, menorrhagia (b) menorrhagia

Fig. 4.13 Features and symptoms of dysfunctional uterine bleeding.

insufficiency. It is commonly associated with infertility.

(iv) *Prolonged corpus luteum activity.* This is extremely rare and occurs as a result of persistent progesterone production in the absence of pregnancy and results in either prolonged periods or protracted episodes of menstrual bleeding.

Dysfunctional bleeding associated with anovulation

Most instances of anovulatory bleeding are due to abnormal fluctuations in progesterone and oestrogen levels causing acyclical oestrogen withdrawal bleeding or oestrogen breakthrough bleeding. The most clearly defined case of cyclical anovular bleeding is metropathia haemorrhagia (Schroeder's disease) (Fig. 4.14). This

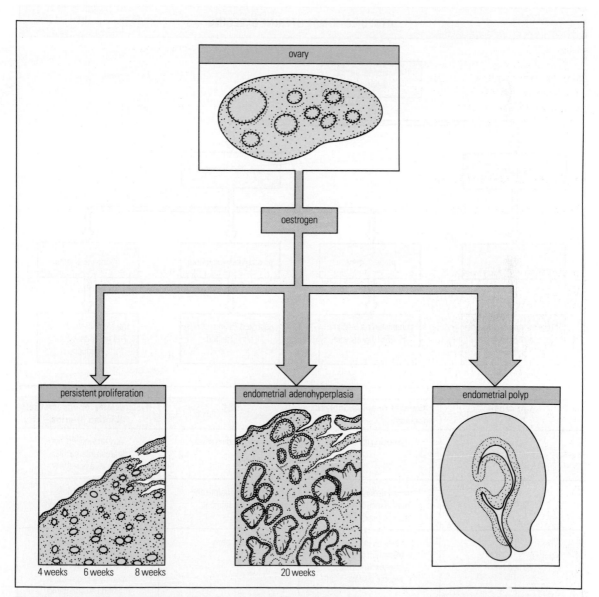

Fig. 4.14 Metropathia haemorrhagia. Diagrammatic illustration of the effects of prolonged oestrogen stimulation on the endometrium of the uterus.

occurs early in the post-puberty and pre-menopausal age groups.

It is characterized by:

(i) Absence of any corpus luteum, active or recent in the ovaries;

(ii) Follicular cysts in one or both ovaries;

(iii) Slight hypertrophy of the uterine muscle;

(iv) Polypoidal hyperplasia of the endometrium;

(v) Characteristic endometrial histology (Swiss cheese endometrium). This is due to prolonged oestrogen stimulation causing endometrial hypertrophy associated with a variable length of amenorrhoea followed by a heavy loss when the oestrogen level falls.

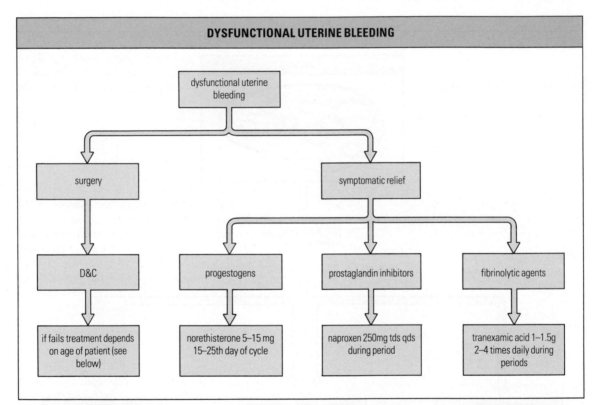

Age range	Hormone or antifibrinolytic therapy	D&C	Hysterectomy or endometrial ablation Uterine
Under 20 years	if bleeding excessive	only if bleeding severe	very rare indeed, but ligation internal iliac arteries a possibility
20-40 years	only if no suspicion of malignancy or for 3 months maximum	preferable before any medical treatment	infrequent and only after all other methods fail
40 and over	never as initial treatment and only after exclusion of organic disease	obligatory	frequenctly if recurrent bleeding and failure of D&C and hormone therapy. ? Endometrial oblation an alternative

Fig. 4.15 Management of dysfunctional uterine bleeding.

One may also find adenomatous hyperplasia of the endometrium thought by some to be pre-cancerous.

Other types of anovulatory bleeding include 'threshold bleeding', i.e. the endometrium is under oestrogen influence, but is thin and poorly developed.

Management of dysfunctional uterine bleeding

The management of dysfunctional uterine bleeding is dependant on the age of the patient (Fig. 4.15). Abnormal uterine bleeding in women younger than 35 years tends to be due to anovulatory bleeding and the likelihood of malignancy is small. In girls under 20 years of age, the cause is usually dysfunctional and undergoes spontaneous cure. If the bleeding is troublesome, menstrual control by hormone therapy is beneficial. In the reproductive era one must bear in mind the possibility of

a complication of early pregnancy as the cause. Biopsy of the endometrium is indicated in all women under 35 if medical treatment fails or the dysfunctional bleeding recurs.

In women over 35 years of age, and certainly over the age of 40, an organic lesion is the most common cause. It is therefore necessary to carry out a diagnostic curettage (or endometrial biopsy as an outpatient) to detect endometrial hyperplasia or intrauterine malignancy. A hysteroscopy with direct visualization of the endometrial cavity can be helpful in cases of persistent or recurrent uterine bleeding. If hormonal therapy is used then the patient should be carefully followed up. If this fails or is contraindicated or the patient's life style is being disrupted by the bleeding, a hysterectomy may be indicated.

Special categories of bleeding

Post-menopausal bleeding
Post-menopausal bleeding should be assumed to be caused by malignancy until proven otherwise (Fig. 4.16). This means excluding benign or malignant lesions of the lower part of the urinary tract and rectum as well as the genital tract. In these cases a diagnostic curettage is mandatory with cystoscopy to exclude urethral and bladder lesions and sigmoidoscopy to rule out lesions of the rectum.

Post-coital bleeding
Post-coital bleeding can occur as a result of a benign cervical or vaginal lesion, but may also be due to a malignant lesion. Post-coital bleeding is often a relatively late symptom in carcinoma of the cervix because the lesion starts in the deeper layers of the epidermis and bleeding cannot occur until the superficial epithelium has been broken through. At the same time extension of the carcinoma occurs into the dermis.

Intermenstrual bleeding
Intermenstrual bleeding is regarded by most women as abnormal even though it may be related to ovulation bleeding. In the premenopausal era of life a carcinoma of the endometrium can give rise to intermenstrual bleeding and the diagnosis should be excluded in women aged 40 and over.

CAUSES OF POST MENOPAUSAL BLEEDING OTHER THAN UTERINE

Cervical lesions

neoplasia, benign and malignant
polyps,
carcinoma

Vaginal lesions

carcinoma, sarcoma or adenosis, laceration or trauma
coital injury, infections, foreign bodies, pessaries, vaginal
adhesions, atrophic vaginitis

Bleeding from other sites

urinary tract and urethra
urethral caruncle

gastrointestinal tract and rectum

external genitalia
labial varices, candylomas, labial trauma, inflammation,
neoplasia, benign and malignant, vulval dystrophy and
atrophic conditions

Fig. 4.16 Causes of post-menopausal bleeding other than uterine.

In general, post-menopausal and intermenstrual bleeding will be reported earlier by the patient than post-coital bleeding. All three symptoms may be a symptom of malignancy of the genital tract and require investigation to establish the cause of the abnormal bleeding.

DYSMENORRHOEA

Dysmenorrhoea is the occurrence of pelvic pain at, or about, the time of menstruation which is sufficiently severe enough to interfere with the work of the patient (most women have some discomfort).

It is now accepted that most menstrual pain is caused by the production of prostaglandins by the uterus. Other symptoms associated with menstruation, such as diarrhoea, headache, nausea and vomiting, are probably also due to prostaglandins. These symptoms can be alleviated by drugs that inhibit prostaglandin synthesis. Various types of dysmenorrhoea are described. Primary (spasmodic) dysmenorrhoea is uterine in origin and very common in girls between 16 and 21. So-called 'secondary dysmenorrhoea' arises outside the uterus, but its association with menstruation is related to the pelvic blood supply and pelvic congestion. It is of great importance to take an accurate history of the pain, paying particular attention to the age of onset, its site, radiation, character, duration, time of onset in relation to menstruation (Fig. 4.17), time of maximum severity and any related symptoms.

Primary (uterine) dysmenorrhoea

Primary dysmenorrhoea (also termed spasmodic, true, intrinsic, functional or essential dysmenorrhoea). The pain arises from the uterus and is related to muscle contractions. It commences with the onset of menstruation or a few hours before and rarely lasts, in severe form, for longer than one day. The pain is felt in the suprapubic region and often radiates to the inner aspects of the thighs and to the back. It may be associated with nausea, vomiting, fainting, diarrhoea, frequency of micturition, dysuria, rectal tenesmus. Severe spasmodic dysmenorrhoea does not usually arise until two or three years after the menarche, as for the first year or two the cycles are usually anovular. This type of dysmenorrhoea only occurs in ovulatory cycles.

There are several theories proposed concerning the aetiology of the symptom, these include: cervical obstruction, uterine hypoplasia, hormonal factors, myometrial factors, innervation factors and uterine prostaglandin production. It is possible that uterine muscle ischaemia related to uterine contractions are important, but recent work has implicated the local activity of prostaglandins to be the most likely cause. Nevertheless, the symptoms are also prone to exaggeration by family, social and psychological factors.

Treatment consists of general health measures, education of the patient and more specific approaches. For mild cases, simple non-narcotic analgesics may suffice. Antispasmodics will give relief, but are not reliable. More specific treatments include non-steroidal anti-prostaglandins and suppression of ovulation with an oral combined oestrogen and progestogen preparation which gives the best results. There is no indication or justification nowadays for cervical dilatation, and presacral neurectomy and alcohol injections of the pelvic plexus are not recommended methods of treatment.

Other variations of uterine dysmenorrhoea include:

(i) Dysmenorrhoea associated with passages of clots.

(ii) Membranous dysmenorrhoea where the whole endometrium is shed as a complete cast of the uterus. This is not generally a recurrent condition.

(iii) Dysmenorrhoea associated with congenital malformations of the uterus. This is particularly found where there is an unequal development of the double genital tract.

(iv) Dysmenorrhoea, associated with uterine pathology. For example with adenomyosis the increased size of the uterus and the presence of more fibrous tissue in the uterine muscle interferes with the normal contractibility of uterine muscle. A fibroid polyp may cause pain if it is extruded through the cervical canal and cervical disease or trauma, although this rarely produces dysmenorrhoea, it may not be taken into account because of the presence of other symptoms such as abnormal bleeding.

Secondary (extrauterine) dysmenorrhoea

Extrauterine or secondary dysmenorrhoea is often regarded as a congestive type of dysmenorrhoea compared with primary dysmenorrhoea for which the cause is principally of uterine aetiology. There is a diffuse, dull ache in the pelvis which is often associated with low backache, especially where there is a pre-existing back problem, however minor. Pre-menstrual engorgement of the pelvis occurs, commencing two or three days prior to menstruation. The pain builds up to be relieved by the onset of menstruation and relief of engorgement.

This dysmenorrhoea is often associated with chronic pelvic sepsis such as salpingo-oophoritis. Other causes are illustrated in Fig. 4.18. Surgery is often required although antibiotics and heat treatment to the pelvis should be tried first.

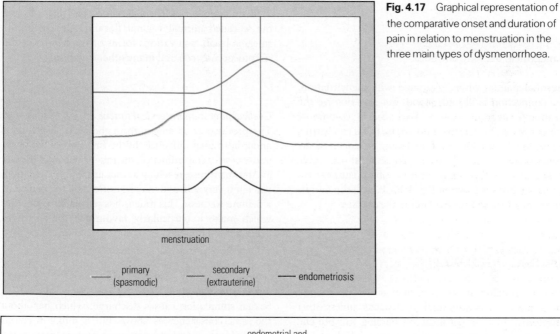

Fig. 4.17 Graphical representation of the comparative onset and duration of pain in relation to menstruation in the three main types of dysmenorrhoea.

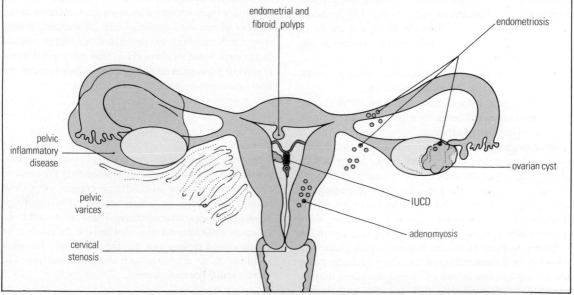

Fig. 4.18 Some of the common causes of secondary dysmenorrhoea.

Dysmenorrhoea associated with endometriosis

The ectopic endometrium responds to hormonal stimulation, becoming engorged prior to menstruation giving rise to a dull pain which worsens as menstruation occurs since the ectopic endometrium bleeds into itself and surrounding tissues. Treatment is that of the endometriosis, either hormonal or surgical or a combination of both.

Management of dysmenorrhoea

Intestinal pain is often associated with menstruation. The connection is ill-understood, but may involve the autonomic nervous system. Backache is commonly thought to be of gynaecological origin, this is rarely true, but certainly any pre-existing lesion is worsened by pelvic congestion and the pain becomes most noticeable at that time. A flow chart of a possible treatment for dysmenorrhoea is given in Fig. 4.19. Pelvic pain and its causes are discussed further later in the chapter.

VAGINAL DISCHARGE

Women complaining of a vaginal discharge are not always aware it is abnormal in character unless other symptoms, such as pruritus or burning are present. There are three levels in the amount of discharge which ordinarily occur during the life of a woman:

(i) pre-puberty, there is only enough to maintain the normal moistness of the vaginal tract;
(ii) after puberty, and particularly during sexual maturity there is an added discharge;
(iii) after pregnancy, there is apt to be a still greater amount of discharge as a result of laceration of the cervix or of cervicitis.

Since many women become accustomed successively to these three different levels, they are not always aware of any change in the amount or character of the discharge that might accompany the onset of pathogenic infestation or infection. So they may only seek advice when, for them, it seems excessive, for example: there is noticeable staining of their underwear; there is an offensive, unpleasant odour; if there is also irritation or soreness, or if there is a suspicion of the discharge being blood stained. The causes of vaginal discharge may be classified as (a) physiological and (b) pathological (Fig. 4.20).

Physiological causes of vaginal discharge

The cervical secretion which maintains the normal moistness of the vagina, is rarely a cause of complaint unless it is profuse. The vagina has no mucus glands and, hence the term 'vaginal mucosa' is a misnomer.

The first type of normal secretion is a clear, mucous discharge with the general consistency of egg white. It is made up largely of mucus in which are found a moderate number of leucocytes and epithelial cells and the so-called normal vaginal flora: Doderlein bacilli, smegma bacilli and various forms of staphylococci and streptococci, *E. coli* and many other organisms.

Cyclical alteration in cervical mucus
The production of mucus from the cervical glands is under hormonal influence. In the first half of the cycle, under oestrogenic influence, the mucus becomes thinner and more profuse, reaching a peak just before ovulation, when it is very thin and may be noticed by the patient as a definite wetness. This mucus has particular properties which make it particularly favourable for sperm to penetrate.

Sexual stimulation
Sexual stimulation causes discharge, which has about the same consistency as above, but is milky in colour and under the microscope shows a great increase in the number of cornified epithelial cells. It contains similar types and numbers of organisms to those already mentioned. Some workers claim that the vaginal secretion is not a secretion at all, but a transudate through the skin (squamous epithelium) of the vagina.

Pregnancy
Pregnancy will increase the activity of all the sexual glands and excessive discharge is frequently the cause of complaint. This type of discharge consists of a clear, transparent mucus, in which are found white lumps having the appearance of curds. These are found to be collections of cornified epithelial cells; if the curds were evenly mixed throughout the fluid portion, the result would be milky discharge such as the second type. The usual vaginal flora are present.

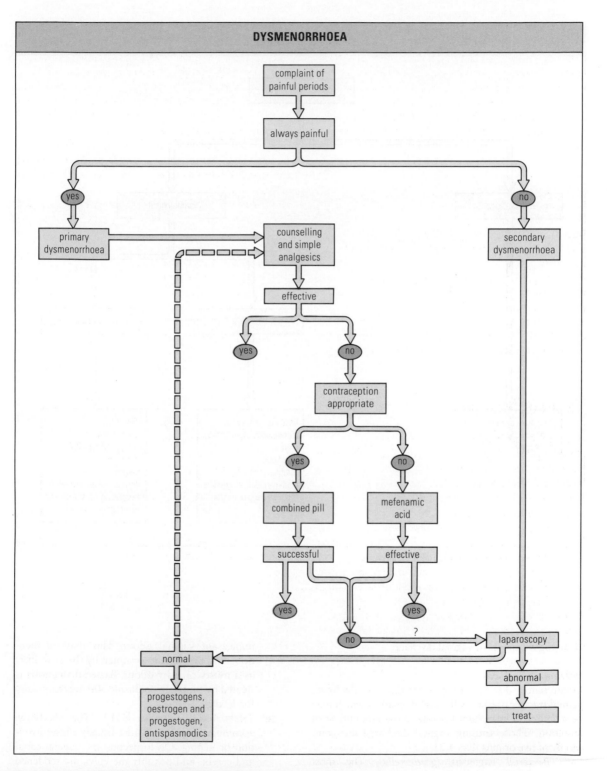

Fig. 4.19 Suggested management of dysmenorrhoea.

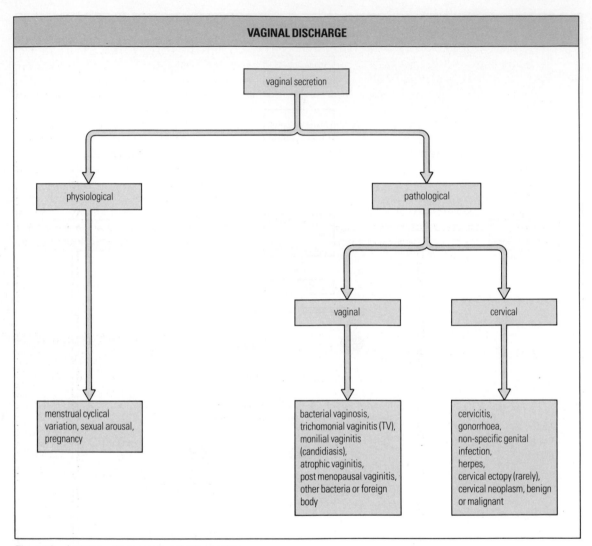

Fig. 4.20 Aetiology of increased vaginal secretion.

Pathological causes of vaginal discharge

Inflammatory diseases

Inflammatory diseases of any of the glands of the lower genital tract or urethra will cause discharges which may be a source of complaint because of the amount, or of irritation. Those causing vaginal discharge are commonly of five origins (Fig. 4.21):

(i) *Bacterial vaginosis (gardnerella).* The most noticeable symptom of this infection is an unpleasant vaginal odour. This may be mentioned by the patient (or noted by the examiner) as a musty or fishy odour. Bacterial vaginosis is treated by oral metronidazole 500 mg twice daily for 10 days.

(ii) *Trichomonal vaginitis (TV).* The discharge accompanying this disorder usually causes irritation or itching. On inspection the vaginal canal and cervix, and possibly the vulva are reddened and appear inflamed. In severe infections there may be haemorrhagic spots on the vaginal mucosa. In milder infections the discharge differs little from normal except that it is slightly more green to yellow in colour and contains more pus cells. With severe infections the discharge is distinctly purulent and often contains small air bubbles (because this protozoal organism is partly anaerobic). The treatment is metronidazol 200 mg three times daily for 7–10 days and the sexual partner should also be treated.

(iii) *Monilial vaginitis (candidiasis)*. In contrast to TV, monilialiasis presents a greyish and congested vaginal mucosa with masses of caseous matter (like cream cheese) which tends to adhere to the mucosa of the vagina and cervix. Severe irritation is often present and may be excruciating. Monilial infection is probably the most common of the known causes of pruritus vulvae (see below). Diabetes mellitus is a predisposing factor and monialiasis is also more likely to be found in pregnancy. The presence of *Candida albicans* in the vagina, especially if accompanied by vulvitus, is said to be an important source of thrush infection for the newborn.

A variety of treatments are available for vulvo-vaginal candidiasis. One of the earliest to be used and still available is aqueous gentian violet, although nystatin pessaries or cream, clotrimazole, miconazole and other agents are more commonly used nowadays.

(iv) *Cervicitis*. Discharge from cervicitis is usually clear to whitish, mucoid or yellow mucopurulent and best treated by cryosurgery, electrocautery or diathermy.

VAGINAL DISCHARGE					
	Discharge at introitus	Symptom	Presence in vagina	Colour	Treatment
Normal	no	none	vault	white	
Bacterial vaginosis (gardnerella)	yes	odour	adherent to vaginal wall	greyish white	metronidazole
Trichomonas vaginalis (TV)	yes	discharge	adherent to vaginal wall	yellowish green with bubbles	metronidazole
Monilia (candida) infections	no	pruritus	adherent to vaginal wall	white	anti-fungal preparations (imidazoles orally)
Cervicitis	minimal	discharge	cervix	clear to whitish	cryosurgery, electrocautery or diathermy
Atrophic vaginitis	no	burning on micturition	vagina (+ vulval atrophy)	red or white	oestrogen cream

Fig. 4.21 Summary diagram of the main pathological causes of vaginal discharge.

(v) *Atrophic vaginitis.* This mild inflammation, which is aggravated by invasion of the mucosa by organisms of low virulence commonly found in the vagina, may produce a discharge which causes a burning sensation, particularly on micturition and often pruritus vulvae. The discharge is usually watery and whitish, but may be bloodstained as a result of the breakdown of adhesions. Best treated by local oestrogen cream or hormone replacement therapy, if appropriate.

Discharge may also be present in gonorrhoea, but is considered in a later chapter.

Other causes

Symptoms that suggest a cervical infection will include vaginal discharge along with deep dyspareunia and post-coital bleeding. *Chlamydia trachomatis* is the major aetiological agent in women with mucopurulent cervicitis. Pelvic inflammation, tumours or cysts are said to cause increased glandular activity and discharge. Venous congestion in the pelvis from any cause may result in vaginal discharge. Clinical conditions include cystic and solid tumours of the uterus, ovary, tube, broad ligaments, relaxation of the pelvic floor from lacerations, over-stretching, cystocele or rectocele and displacement of the uterus following retroversion and prolapse. The discharge is of normal appearance.

Ulceration

Ulceration of any sort causes discharge because of exudations from the ulcerated surface. Such ulcerations result from syphilis and other sexually transmitted diseases, tuberculosis, erosion of the cervix, ulceration in malignant lesions, chemical or mechanical trauma and unhealed lacerations of childbirth. The discharge may be distinctly serous or it may be indistinguishable from that of other causes. It is frequently blood stained.

Management of vaginal discharges

In all pathological discharges the cause has to be diagnosed by taking swabs for culture including using special transporting media. Having established a cause then appropriate treatment can be given as indicated earlier. If a specific cause is not identified then the treatment is largely empirical with antibiotics, anti-fungal preparations or metronidazole.

It is important to remember that approximately 25% of trichomonal and monilial infections are asymptomatic and that oral broad spectrum antibiotics are often associated with the development of monilial infections.

PRURITUS VULVAE

Pruritus means a sensation of itching. It is important to determine whether the pruritus is truly vulval because it can also be vaginal or anal. Indeed it may merely be one part of a generalized dermatological problem. A summary of the main causes of pruritus vulvae is shown in Fig. 4.22.

Causes

Pruritus associated with vaginal discharge

Trichomonas vaginalis or *Candida albicans* account for about 80% of all cases of pruritus vulvae of recent onset.

Pruritus without vaginal discharge

This accounts for 15–20% of the causes and is a most difficult clinical problem. It may be part of a generalized pruritus, e.g. jaundice or Hodgkin's disease. Since the vulval area is hair-bearing it may be infested with organisms such as scabies. Squamous cell carcinoma of the vulva may cause itching in the early stage. Carcinoma *in situ* and Paget's disease of the vulva can cause pruritus for many years before becoming invasive.

Parasitic infections

These infections affect the pubic area, but may also involve the vulva.

Diseases of the anus and rectum

These diseases are often related to monilia. Occasionally conditions of the urinary tract may cause soreness because of chafing, but rarely cause pruritus. The only common cause is glycosuria whether associated with diabetes mellitus or low renal threshold.

Allergy and drug sensitivity
An allergy is often a cause, especially if one thinks of all the chemicals which may be applied to the area, e.g. soaps, talc etc., clothing materials or even nail varnish on the patient's fingers. Sometimes there is sensitivity to contraceptives i.e. rubber in the barrier methods (condoms or diaphragms) or chemical materials used.

Deficiency states
An example of this is avitaminosis or the presence of achlorhydria.

Physiological factors
Physiological factors are more often contributory factors rather than the primary cause.

Chronic epithelial dystrophies
These are not uncommon, particularly atrophic changes noted in the post-menopausal woman.

Management of pruritus vulvae
A thorough history should be taken to ensure the proper identification and management of the disorder. Enquiries should be made about the use of any hormones, topical applications or medicines and about home remedies such as local anaesthetics and ointments. Many patients use self treatments for the vulva in the hope that the symptom will go away without needing to consult their doctor or a gynaecologist. Self applied medications may improve, aggravate or alter the appearance of any lesions present and interfere in making the correct diagnosis. Other important points are menstrual and sexual habits, methods of contracep-

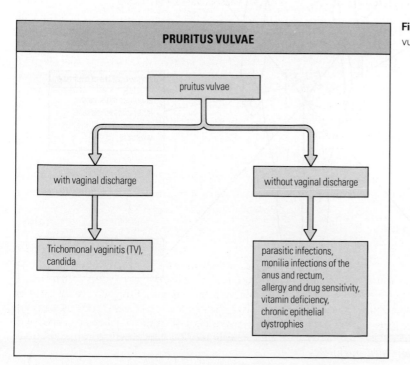

Fig. 4.22 Major causes of pruritus vulvae.

tion, response to previous treatment(s) and a history of allergy.

Each case requires careful investigation since pruritus vulvae is only a symptom. Diagnosis and treatment is relatively easy when the pruritus is accompanied by a vaginal discharge (see previous section). When no cause can be found, then the treatment is empirical and often proves unsatisfactory. With proper investigation and treatment, cure or relief can be obtained in the majority of cases.

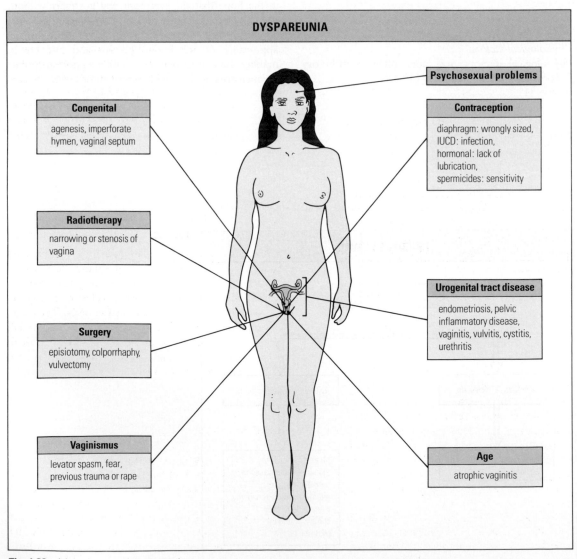

Fig. 4.23 Major causes of dyspareunia.

DYSPAREUNIA

Painful sexual intercourse is usually classified as superficial or deep. These respectively reflect (i) causes related at or near the entrance or lower part of the vagina and (ii) those at the cervix, vault of the vagina or pelvic area. Sexual intercourse is not normally painful. However, every sexually active woman probably has occasional discomfort from lack of lubrication, prolonged coital contact or minor genital disorders. Slight pain may occur, but not be considered a problem if it does not interfere with desire, arousal or orgasm. As a gynaecological symptom it is related to those who present with pain or it may be elicited during the course of the history taking. Some of the possible causes of dyspareunia are given in Fig. 4.23.

Superficial dyspareunia

Superficial causes of dyspareunia include any skin lesions, but in particular Bartholin's abscess. Also severe vaginal and vulval infection with monilia which is often accompanied by a complaint of pruritus vulvae. Any laceration or overenthusiastic embroidery (e.g. repair of episiotomy or posterior repair) may cause discomfort. The truly 'imperforate' or rigid hymen and vaginal septum have to be excluded. In many cases the dyspareunia is due to levator spasm. It is important to remember that both levator muscles are attached to the vagina and if contracted form an obstruction about one inch from the vaginal orifice.

Deep dyspareunia

Deep dyspareunia may be related to a retroverted uterus, since the ovaries are attached to the back of the uterus they prolapse into the Pouch of Douglas (like the testes, the ovaries are sensitive if in a fixed position and knocked). A mobile retroversion is present in about one in 10–20 women although only occasionally will dyspareunia occur. It is the fixed retroversion which gives rise to symptoms. The common causes of fixed retroversion are chronic pelvic infection and endometriosis.

Treatment of dyspareunia is of the underlying cause, hence the need for accurate diagnosis. Any examination must be very gentle. If the pain that is experienced during coitus can be reproduced during examination an organic cause must be suspected. It may be necessary to examine the patient under anaesthesia or perform a laparoscopic examination to establish the diagnosis. There may be an underlying psychological or psychosexual problem which complicates the problem. Although organic disease is an important factor 50–60% of women do not have identifiable organic disease present.

Vaginismus

This is recurrent involuntary spasm of the pubococcygeus and levator ani muscles which occurs to interfere or prevent coitus. It is a conditioned reflex for which the provoking stimulus is the previous experience of pain. The management of this problem requires considerable skill and patience on the part of the gynaecologist. Although vaginal dilators may be used they do not cause mechanical dilatation, as the normal introitus does not need stretching, they are to help the woman gain conscious control over the levator muscles and thereby overcome the spasm.

PELVIC PAIN

Pelvic as well as abdominal pain may result from haemorrhage, infection or neoplasm of the internal genitalia or as a complication of pregnancy. It may also have a non-gynaecological origin in the gastrointestinal tract, urinary tract or peritoneum. Pelvic pain may be referred from or to other sites in the body. There are innumerable pathological conditions and functional disorders which, in conjunction with the individual response to pain and pain threshold, makes localization of pain a diagnostic dilemma.

Pelvic nerve supply and pain

Whilst nerve endings extend into all the internal pelvic organs they are few in number. Since there is no great concentration of sensory nerve ganglia in the pelvis the central nervous system cannot easily identify pain that arises from the pelvic organs. This makes it difficult for women to describe and localize their pain. Basically, the sources of pelvic pain are related to distention of a hollow viscus, peritoneal irritation or inflammation or

65

ischaemia of a functioning muscle tissue.

Visceral abdominal pain tends to be poorly localized because sensory impulses from the pelvic and abdominal viscera overlap within the same segment of the spinal cord. Sensations from pelvic organs are transmitted by three pathways. (i) The parasympathetic nerves (S2, S3 and 4) transmit sensation to the spinal cord via the hypogastric plexus from the upper third of the vagina up to the lower uterine segment, the posterior urethra, the trigone, lower ureters, the uterosacral and cardinal ligaments. (ii) The sympathetic nerves (T11, T12 and L1) transmit impulses to the spinal cord via the hypogastric and inferior mesenteric plexuses, from the upper part of the uterus, proximal third of the Fallopian tubes and broad ligaments, the upper part of the bladder and caecum and terminal large bowel. (iii) The superior mesenteric plexus (T5 to T11) transmit impulses to the spinal cord from the ovaries, lateral two thirds of the Fallopian tubes and the upper ureters.

Investigations

As pelvic pain is difficult to describe it is important that a meticulous history is taken. The onset, location, quality, duration and severity of the pain should be considered as well as any associated complaints or symptoms. The sudden onset of pain suggests an acute problem such as perforation, haemorrhage, torsion or rupture, whereas a gradual onset suggests inflammation, obstruction or a slowly evolving problem. Of the associated symptoms, vaginal bleeding is usually associated with pelvic pain and indicates genital tract pathology. Pyrexia and fever are symptomatic of pelvic infection. Anorexia, nausea and vomiting are non-specific and indicate intestinal tract pathology. Fainting, collapse and shock usually suggest intraperitoneal bleeding, secondary to hypovolaemia. Symptoms which indicate urinary tract pathology are dysuria, polyuria and frequency (discussed further in Chapter 7, Gynaeological Urology). Primary dysmenorrhoea and secondary dysmenorrhoea are separate entities which have already been described. Dyspareunia, which has several aetiologies, has also been described separately.

A history of ectopic pregnancy increases the risk of a subsequent ectopic. A history of chronic pelvic inflammatory disease increases the risk of an acute exacerbation of a chronic problem and for the possibility of an ectopic pregnancy.

A physical examination must include a general examination, abdominal, pelvic and rectal examination,

even though the latter two may be uncomfortable. Of additional investigations, ultrasound may be useful for evaluating the pelvic organs, the diagnosis of an early intrauterine pregnancy, a molar pregnancy or an ovarian mass. Laparoscopy is the most useful investigative tool for the assessment of obscure pelvic pain not accurately localized by detailed examination.

In the majority of cases a normal pelvis will be found in about 30% of women, pelvic inflammatory disease in 25%, ovarian or pelvic pathology in about 25–30% of cases and a residual group which will consist of pelvic congestion, uterine fibroids, endometriosis or ectopic pregnancy. The common causes of pelvic pain are depicted in Fig. 4.24.

Causes

Acute pelvic pain

With acute pain the patient typically seeks medical advice promptly and certain diagnoses should always be considered. Namely, pregnancy related conditions, abortion and ectopic pregnancy, gynaecological conditions such as salpingitis, torsion or rupture of an ovarian cyst and endometriosis. Non-gynaecological causes will include appendicitis, pyelonephritis, renal calculus, intestinal obstruction, diverticulitis and other bowel disease. An awareness of the type of contraception used is also valuable. Salpingitis and ectopic pregnancy are more common amongst users of intrauterine devices than with women who take oral contraceptives.

Chronic pelvic pain

Some causes of chronic pain and their characteristics are given in Fig. 4.25. It is important that in the investigation of chronic pelvic pain the patient should be asked 'what did you do when the pain started?' as well as 'what do you do that makes the pain better or worse?'

Psychosomatic disease

When there is obvious pathology and confirmatory evidence of a cause the interpretation of pelvic pain is easy. However, when no abnormalities exist or when pelvic pain and associated symptoms seem to be out of proportion to the physical findings the evaluation and treatment is much more confusing. The patient is usually very vague in her description of her pain and a distinction between functional and organic causes is more difficult. In addition to having pelvic symptomatology, which may include vaginismus, dyspareunia, abnormal vaginal bleeding and urinary frequency the patient almost invariably has many associated general symptoms of dizziness, headaches, weakness, fatigue, depression, nausea and vomiting. The symptoms being aggravated by a menstrual cycle. There seems to be an

acceptance that pelvic pain can be due to a functional cause related to some form of emotional disorder. Yet in some women the symptoms are related to pelvic congestion and so ligation of the venous supply improves the problem. No woman should be labelled as having psychosomatic pelvic pain until all possible causes have been excluded.

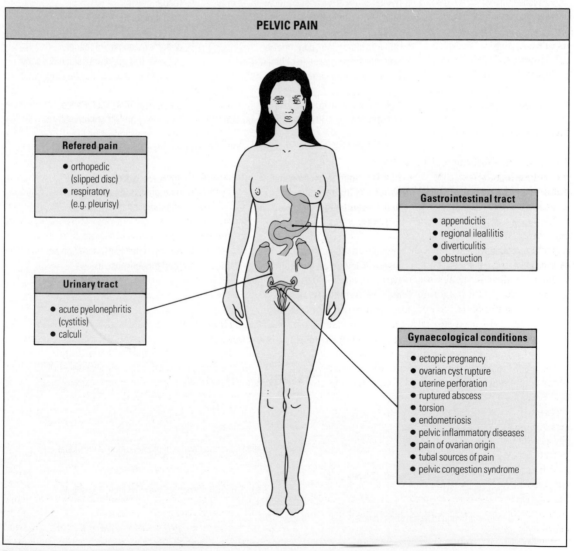

Fig. 4.24 Common causes of pelvic pain.

CHRONIC PELVIC PAIN		
Diagnosis	History	Physical examination
Endometriosis	dysmenorrhoea, dyspareunia, infertility, prolonged menses	tender pelvis; uterosacral nodularity; adnexal masses; fixed retroversion of uterus
Chronic pelvic inflammatory disease	history of acute salpingitis, bilateral lower abdominal pain, menorrhagia, dysmenorrhoea, dyspareunia	tender pelvis; tender pelvic masses
Psychosomatic disorders	dyspareunia often associated with anxiety, depression and other systemic complaints	tender pelvis; no palpable pathology
Chronic diverticulitis	dull left-sided pain, constipation and diarrhoea, passage of blood and mucus, older age	abdomen and pelvis tender in lower left quadrant; signoidoscopy and barium enema may be diagnostic
Regional enteritis	right-sided pain, diarrhoea or constipation, blood in stool, younger age	chronically ill in appearance; mass may be felt abdominally or on pelvic examination; x-ray studies diagnostic
Functional bowel disease	pain is related to position and action e.g. lifting, standing and is not related to menses, fertility or coitus	left lower quadrant tenderness; improves with antispasmodic medication
Musculoskeletal disorder	cramping abdominal pain mostly in lower left quadrant with no relationship to menses, fertility or coitus; passage of mucus with stool	resuts of pelvic examination normal; tender back muscles

Fig. 4.25 Some causes of chronic pelvic pain and their presenting characteristics.

HIRSUTISM

End result of:

1 number of hair follicles

2 degree in which androgens affect types of hair (in male areas)

3 ratio of growing to resting hair follicle

4 thickness and degree of pigmentation of individual hairs

5 asynchrony of growth cycles in aggregates of hair follicles

Fig. 4.26 Factors affecting hair distribution.

Management of pelvic pain

In general, chronic pelvic pain is usually associated with pelvic pathology and the appropriate treatment can be given. Where there is no obvious cause one should start by giving the patient analgesics or antispasmodics to render her as symptom-free as possible. Whatever drugs are chosen they should be reduced gradually as she begins to respond to reassurance and supportive therapy which may have to be given over several months.

HIRSUTISM

Hirsutism indicates the presence of excessive hair with or without signs of virilization. Hair is excessive when its growth is more profuse or longer in a given site than is the norm for an individual's age, race and sex (Figs 4.26 and 4.27). Hair distribution is essentially similar in men and women, but the differences are due mainly to the different level of circulating androgens. The possibility of abnormal hairiness in women always exist and when present can be a significant emotional, psychological and cosmetic problem for the patient. It may be accompanied by anovulatory amenorrhoea, dysfunctional uterine bleeding or infertility. Virilization involves hirsuitism accompanied by increased muscle mass, clitoralomegaly, voice deepening and increased libido. There may also be signs of defeminization such as decreased breast size and loss of vaginal lubrication.

Causes

Numerous factors can cause hirsutism including endocrinological causes and non endocrinological causes. Hirsutism alone, in the absence of signs of virilization is usually associated with very mild androgen excess and target organ (hair follicle) sensitivity. Isolated hirsutism is often also due to genetic, idiopathic or racial factors. Genetic factors are important in sexual hair growth regulation, as demonstrated in siblings, familial generations or ethnic groups.

Investigations

The cause of the patient's hirsutism may be determined by taking a detailed history and a genetic or familial factor elicited. The patient should be particularly questioned about signs of virilization such as menstrual irregularities, infertility, alopecia, deepening of the voice, increased muscle mass and clitoral enlargement. Possible iatrogenic causes related to drug therapy

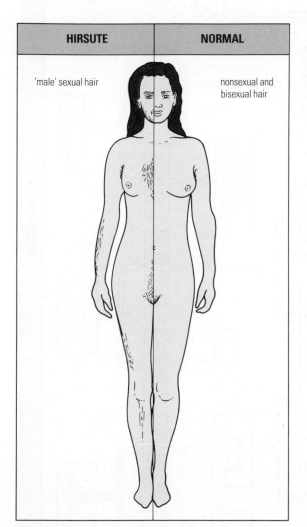

HIRSUTE	NORMAL
'male' sexual hair	nonsexual and bisexual hair

Fig. 4.27 Comparison of hair distribution in the normal and hirsute female. The distribution of hair is under hormonal control: nonsexual hair by growth hormone from the pituitary; bisexual hair by low levels of androgens produced by the ovaries in the female, and the male pattern by a high concentration of androgens.

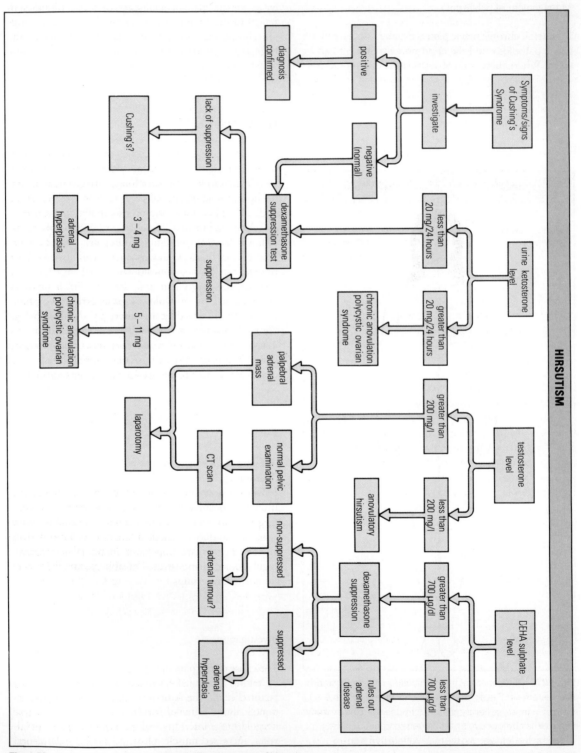

Fig. 4.28 A possible scheme for establishing the cause of hirsutism.

should be checked. During examination the doctor must assess whether hirsutism really exists or whether the patient had just become aware of slightly excessive hair growth. The physical signs of virilization mentioned above should be looked for and special care to note any signs of adrenal disorders. During the pelvic examination the doctor should search for any adnexal masses bearing in mind that fewer than a third of ovarian androgen secreting tumours are palpable.

The onset of hirsutism, if acute, is often accompanied by signs of virilization as seen by androgen secreting tumours. If of gradual onset and increasing irregularity of the menstrual cycle it may reflect polycystic ovary syndrome.

A wide range of tests are available for determining the cause of hirsutism and the investigations can be on an out-patient or in-patient basis (Fig. 4.28). Bearing in mind that the majority of patients will have idiopathic hirsutism or polycystic ovary syndrome a short admission to evaluate the endocrine systems likely to be involved is appropriate. The majority of cases of severe endocrine disturbance are in fact unlikely to be referred initially to the gynaecologist with hirsutism.

The short stay admission will involve adrenal suppression and stimulation tests, plasma cortisol, plasma testosterone, plasma androstenedione, plasma progesterone and oestradiol, sex hormone binding globulin, FSH, LH and prolactin estimations.

When the results are available the diagnosis of idiopathic hirsutism will be confirmed by exclusion or a particularly abnormal result will identify areas which need detailed investigation. For example, very high androgen levels suggesting a tumour would require further admission for localization of the tumours. Once the results of the investigations are known the requirements for fertility can be considered.

Management of hirsutism

If the diagnosis of hyperprolactinaemia or polycystic ovarian syndrome (POS) is made and fertility is required then appropriate therapy can be commenced. If conception is not required and the diagnosis is POS then ethinyl oestradiol 30 μg for 21 days from day 5 of the menstrual cycle and cyproterone acetate 50 mg from day 15–25 for 6–9 months is appropriate, although therapy may be continued for longer. Sometimes prednisolone 0.5 mg and 0.25 mg morning and evening is given daily as an alternative. Idiopathic hirsutism may be treated similarly if conception is not required.

Local treatments include shaving, electrolysis and depilatory creams, of varying cost and effectiveness.

GALACTORRHOEA

Galactorrhoea is the abnormal breast secretion of milk and can occur in both men and women. In order to differentiate normal lactation in women from galactorrhoea there must be an interval of at least one year after breast feeding or pregnancy. Galactorrhoea may be noted by the woman herself or it may be found on examination. In spite of the possible physiological, pathological or pharmacological causes of galactorrhoea the incidence is only about 1–4% in women. Eighty per cent of these women who present with galactorrhoea also have menstrual disturbances such as amenorrhoea or oligomenorrhoea.

Galactorrhoea is both a symptom and a physical finding, and its presence in women can indicate changes in normal prolactin levels (hyperprolactinemia) (Fig. 4.29). Prolactin is the hormone which is secreted by the anterior lobe of the pituitary gland to induce lactation. Although not all women with galactorrhoea will have raised serum prolactin, its level should be estimated in all women with galactorrhoea.

Causes

Pituitary adenomas
Whilst galactorrhoea alone may not be significant, galactorrhoea in association with amenorrhoea and/or hyperprolactinemia has a definite association with pituitary adenomas. Up to a quarter of women with amenorrhoea and galactorrhoea have prolactinomas. Consequently any woman who has galactorrhoea and amenorrhoea should be investigated thoroughly to detect whether a pituitary tumour is present (see also the previous section on amenorrhoea).

Psychotropic drugs
The most common nonorganic cause of galactorrhoea and menstrual irregularity relates to the use of psychotropic drugs, particularly the phenothiazines. These agents alter normal dopamine receptors in the hypothalamus. This disruption of the dopaminergic neural pathway can result in elevation of the serum prolactin.

71

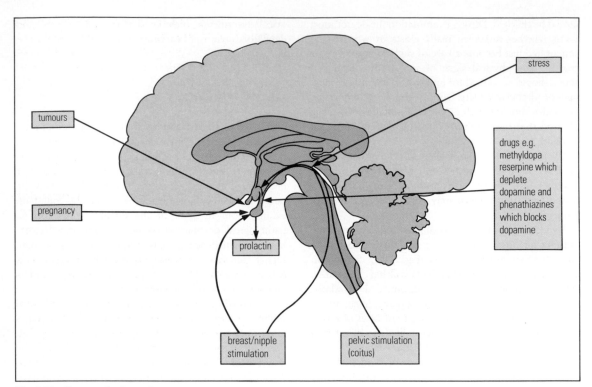

Fig. 4.29 Causes of galactorrhoea.

These drugs also alter normal hypothalamic pituitary gonadotropin function with resultant menstrual irregularities. Even though psychotropic drugs can result in elevated prolactin levels, overt galactorrhoea only occurs in about half of the women taking this type of therapy.

Oral contraceptives

Oral contraceptives can cause galactorrhoea in two separate ways. The effect of oestrogen and progesterone in oral contraceptives may result in maturation of the breast such that normal prolactin levels may stimulate milk secretion. Coincidentally, oestrogen can increase serum prolactin levels by a direct action. The summation of these two actions may result in overt galactorrhoea, which usually is first noticed by the woman while she is menstruating, as a consequence of stopping the 'pill'. The prolactin effect on the breast is usually blocked by the exogenous steroids during their administration.

Menstrual dysfunction with galactorrhoea and hyperprolactinemia

The menstrual dysfunction that accompanies the elevated serum prolactin levels is probably related to a hypothalamic dysfunction but the exact aetiology is unknown. No clear cut FSH or LH response can be found between hyperprolactinemic women both with or without evidence of a pituitary adenoma. Basal gonadotropin levels, although within the normal range in women with hyperprolactinemia, do show a significant increase in the mean FSH levels during bromocriptine therapy, which inhibits prolactin secretion. Thus indicates that there may be a 'threshold-level' of FSH necessary to stimulate normal ovarian folliculogenesis which is not reached with hyperprolactinemia.

Investigations

It has been found that the prolactin levels do not always

correlate with the presence or absence of a pituitary adenoma, although peripheral prolactin levels greater than 200 ng/ml are highly suspicious for pituitary adenoma. Therefore the pituitary fossa (sella turcica) must be evaluated by radiological methods. Computerized axial tomography (CT) is best reserved for those who have abnormalities of the sella turcica, to exclude supratentorial extension of the tumour, and for large (> 1.0 cm) intrasellar lesions. The newer generation of CT scanners appears to be able to discriminate intrapituitary lesions smaller than 1.0 cm in diameter, but this equipment is not readily available. Formal visual field determinations are used initially to exclude optic chias-

ma compression and are worthwhile for interval evaluations to reduce the exposure to X-rays. Thyroid function studies and TSH levels are standard in the evaluation of hyperprolactinemia. Fig. 4.30 illustrates a possible pattern investigation of patients with galactorrhoea.

Management of galactorrhoea

Treatment of galactorrhoea is of the underlying cause ie. surgery if a pituitary tumour is found, cessation of the use of psychotropic drugs etc. Prolactin levels can be

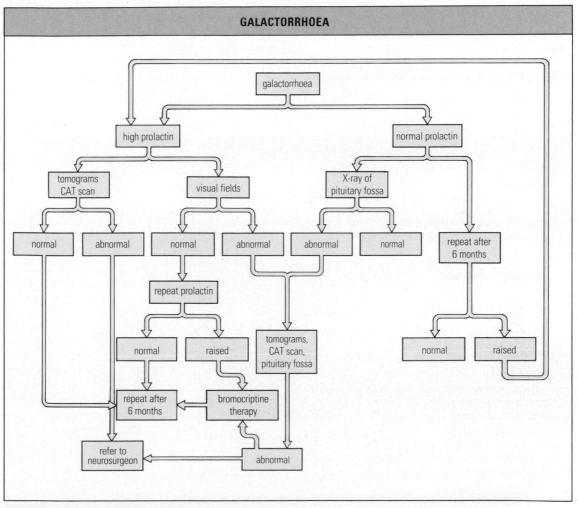

Fig. 4.30 Follow-up of patients with galactorrhoea.

reduced directly by bromocriptine therapy (2.5 mg three times daily), although side-effects include nausea and giddiness. The therapy should be continued for 6–9 months. Since ovulation may become irregular fertility may be restored by other drugs such as clomiphene.

PREMENSTRUAL TENSION

Premenstrual tension is an accentuation of menstrual symptoms and may be present for 7–10 days before menstruation commences and is relieved by the onset of menstruation. The common complaints are listed in Fig. 4.31. It is very common and may affect up to 75% of women at some time in their life.

Causes

There is evidence of an increase in the extracellular fluid throughout the body. The average premenstrual weight gain in these women is 5lb (normal 1lb) and may be as much as 10 lb. Oedema is associated with sodium retention and may be due to high levels of oestrogen or progesterone. It is most probably only associated with ovular cycles.

Management of premenstrual tension

If troublesome, relief may be offered by supportive psychotherapy, analgesics, vitamin B6, minor tranquillisers, bromocriptine, progesterone, oral diuretic therapy, but it is sometimes necessary to suppress ovulation hormonally to satisfy the patient. The majority of the treatment regimes are unproven by controlled trials, but some are effective in individual patients. A sympathetic approach to the problem and a willingness to try many treatments is necessary.

PREMENSTRUAL TENSION: COMMON SYMPTOMS
Physical
breast tenderness and swelling, abdominal bloating, oedema and weight gain, pelvic discomfort, headache, migraine
Autonomic reactions
dizziness/faintness, cold sweats, nausea/vomiting, hot flushes
Psychological
tension, irritability, depression, insomnia, forgetfulness, loss of concentration

Fig. 4.31 Common symptoms of premenstrual tension.

Gynaecological Conditions

ABORTION AND TERMINATION

The terms abortion and miscarriage are synonymous and are defined as the expulsion of the conceptus from the uterine cavity before the 28th week of gestation. Often the term 'miscarriage' is preferable when talking to patients, as abortion tends to imply a termination. At present, pregnancies ending before 28 weeks are classified as miscarriages unless the fetus is born alive. It is now felt that 24 weeks is a more appropriate date since there have been several fetuses who have survived from 24 weeks' gestation onwards. Recent legislation has indeed changed the legal definition of delivery to after 24 weeks and the definition of stillbirth has changed accordingly.

Abortion may be spontaneous or induced and these form two distinct entities.

Spontaneous

It is thought that about 30 per cent of all pregnancies end as spontaneous abortions. The causes of spontaneous abortion are summarized in Fig. 5.1.

Aetiology of spontaneous abortion

The causes tend to differ in abortions which occur before 12-14 weeks' gestation from those which occur later.

Maternal Factors

Infections

Any acute febrile illness causing pyrexia may precipitate abortion. Specific infections, such as rubella, cytomegalovirus and syphilis, may directly affect the fetus.

Endocrine disorders

Although there is an interrelationship between the different endocrine glands, there is no concrete evidence that abnormalities of any endocrine organ interfere with pregnancy. Disorders associated with abortion are hypothyroidism, poorly controlled diabetes, which has an increased risk of malformation and therefore miscarriage, and possibly progesterone deficiency, although this is highly disputed.

Drugs

Cytotoxic drugs, lead, and quinine may all be toxic and cause miscarriage.

Dietary

Various vitamin deficiencies have been blamed for abortion and malformation. Folic acid deficiency is often said to be a factor, but this is not yet proven.

CAUSES OF SPONTANEOUS ABORTION	
Early (up to 12-14 weeks)	**Late (after 14 weeks)**
chromosomal abnormality uterine anomaly dietary drugs trauma	acute infection incompetent cervix trauma hypertension

Fig. 5.1 Causes of spontaneous abortion, classified according to whether they occur early or late in pregnancy.

Trauma
This is a rare cause of abortion, particularly since the Abortion Act of 1967.

Uterine factors
Congenital anatomical abnormalities and submucous fibroids may interfere with adequate implantation and predispose to abortion. Cervical incompetence is the most common uterine factor, but this is usually associated with late (second trimester) abortions.

Fetal factors
It has been found that a very high percentage (more than 50 per cent) of aborted fetuses have a chromosome abnormality. The earlier the abortion occurs, the more likely it is to be due to chromosome abnormality.

The different types of abortion are shown in Fig. 5.2.

Threatened abortion

In these patients, vaginal bleeding occurs, but there are neither uterine contractions, nor abdominal pain, and the cervix does not dilate. Any vaginal bleeding after conception is regarded as a threatened abortion. Whilst it may be decidual bleeding before 12 weeks' gestation, other lesions may occasionally be responsible, e.g. a cervical polyp, cervical ectopy (erosion), or cervical carcinoma, the last being very rare. If the patient requires admission to hospital, vaginal examination should be performed to look for local causes of bleeding. If the cervix is open on speculum examination, products of conception may be seen extruding from the os, in which case the pregnancy is unlikely to be saved even with the insertion of a cervical suture.

Urinary pregnancy tests remain positive if the trophoblastic tissue is viable but a negative pregnancy test can be inconclusive as the pregnancy may be too early for detection.

Ultrasound examination is useful as it can show whether the patient is pregnant and, is so, whether the pregnancy is viable or not. It may also indicate the presence of a hydatidiform mole and whether the pregnancy is within the uterus.

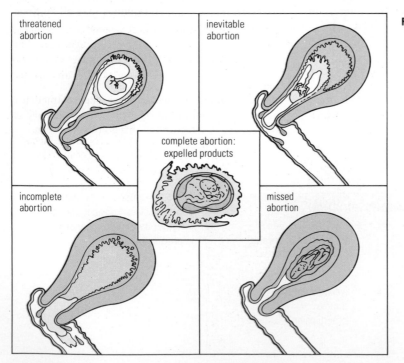

Fig. 5.2 Different types of abortion.

The patient is advised to rest. This does not mean strict bed rest. The patient, however, should stay off work for at least several days. Intercourse should be avoided until bleeding settles. If a viable pregnancy is confirmed, the patient is usually allowed home to rest there. Approximately 90 per cent of threatened miscarriages with a viable pregnancy at 12 weeks will continue to term. At discharge the patient is advised that if the bleeding becomes bright red or is associated with abdominal pain she should be readmitted, as her threatened miscarriage may be becoming inevitable.

Inevitable abortion

When uterine detachments occur and the cervix dilates or the membranes rupture, the pregnancy will inevitably abort. At this'stage, vaginal examination may reveal products of conception protruding through the dilated cervix. Vaginal bleeding is usually heavy. The inevitable abortion may be:

(i) Complete, when the cervix closes and bleeding ceases and no further treatment is required. This is usually the case before eight weeks (before placentation is established) or after 20 weeks (when a miniature labour occurs with expulsion of the fetus and placenta).

(ii) Incomplete, where a variable amount of retained placental tissue causes persistent vaginal bleeding and uterine contractions.

Incomplete abortion is more common than complete abortion. The patient should have an intravenous drip (line) inserted and the evacuation of retained products of conception performed under general anaesthetic, as illustrated in Fig. 5.3. Once this has been done, the uterus will contract down and bleeding will cease. Usually 10 IU of Syntocinon is given to aid the contraction of the uterus.

Missed abortion

This was previously thought to be a relatively rare condition, but the increasing use of early ultrasound scan has increased the diagnosis of missed abortion. It is thought that the chorionic tissue may survive and continue to produce HCG which enables the gestation to remain in the uterus. The patient has a positive pregnancy test, but uterine size is usually smaller than expected, shown in Fig. 5.4. Once the diagnosis is made, treatment depends upon the uterine size: if less than fourteen weeks, curettage or suction curettage is usually performed; if greater than fourteen weeks in size, then it may be appropriate to use oxytocin or prostaglandins. It may be preferable to await spontaneous expulsion of the products of conception as this decreases risk of infection. However, if a conservative approach is used then it is essential to monitor the fibrinogen levels as coagulation defects can occur. These problems, however, are extremely rare before 4 weeks after the demise of the pregnancy. The knowledge by the woman that her pregnancy is no longer viable is usually associated with the desire to have the uterus evacuated.

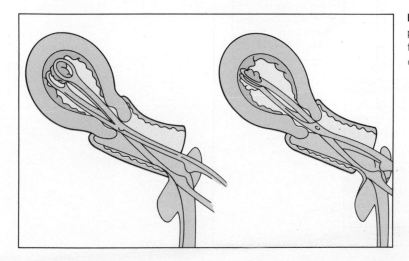

Fig. 5.3 Evacuation of retained products of conception with sponge forceps. This will be followed by curettage of the uterine cavity.

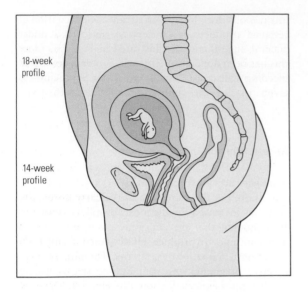

18-week
profile

14-week
profile

Fig. 5.4 Missed abortion of an 18-week pregnancy.

Septic abortion

Any abortion may become infected, especially an incomplete abortion.

Before the Abortion Act, many septic abortions were associated with unskilled attempts to procure abortion with unsterile instruments. The commonest infection organisms are *E. coli* and streptococci. The patient presents pyrexial and toxic, with abdominal pain, and usually offensive vaginal discharge. On examination, the uterus is tender on palpation and in advanced cases there may be signs of peritonitis. Gram negative endotoxic shock may rarely occur and, even more rarely, haemolytic anaemia with *Clostridium welchii* infections may be seen.

Treatment should begin promptly with large doses of broad-spectrum antibiotics such as a cephalosporin and metronidazole. Swabs should be taken from the cervix for culture prior to commencement. The circulation should be maintained. Steriods may be necessary. Fluid balance

Fig. 5.5 Causes of repeated abortion.

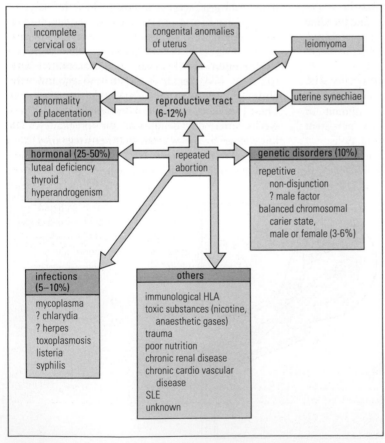

should be carefully observed. Once the infection is under control, the uterus should be emptied under general anaesthetic, but great care is required as the infected uterus is soft and perforation can occur.

Recurrent abortion

This is a sequence of three or more consecutive miscarriages. The possible causes can be divided into congenital and acquired (Fig. 5.5).

Congenital

Congenital causes of recurrent abortion include:

 (i) Chromosome anomalies, particularly balanced translocation of either parent.
 (ii) Uterine anomalies such as partial or complete septums. These can be investigated using a hysterosalpingogram.
 (iii) Cervical anomalies, particularly cervical incompetence, which may be a congenital cause and result in recurrent mid-trimester abortions. A truly incompetent cervix is diagnosed between pregnancies by hysterosalpingogram in the second half of the menstrual cycle, or by observing the easy passage of a 8mm Hegar dilator. Such patients require cervical cerclage in further pregnancies as shown in Fig. 5.6.

Acquired

Acquired causes of recurrent abortions include:

 (i) Trauma: this could be due to excessive dilatation of the cervix during dilatation and curettage or at termination of pregnancy, producing an incompetent cervix in a subsequent pregnancy.
 (ii) Infective: occasionally infections such as cytomegalovirus, listeria or toxoplasmosis can be a cause of recurrent abortions. They need to be excluded, but are uncommon and difficult to treat.
 (iii) Tumour: fibroids in particular may distort the uterine cavity and give rise to recurrent abortions.
 (iv) Hormonal: hyperthyroidism and diabetes have been implicated as potential causes of recurrent abortion, but with appropriate treatment this should be rare. Progesterone deficiency causing recurrent failure of the corpus luteum has been postulated, but there is no hard evidence to support this. Treatment with progesterone seems to be as effective as placebo, but whilst there are many studies that support its use there are an equal number of studies which refute its use.
 (v) Immune causes: there are some cases where the HLA typing between husband and wife shows excessive homozygocity and is associated with recurrent abortions.
 (vi) Poor nutrition or chronic disease, such as renal disease, has been implicated as a factor.

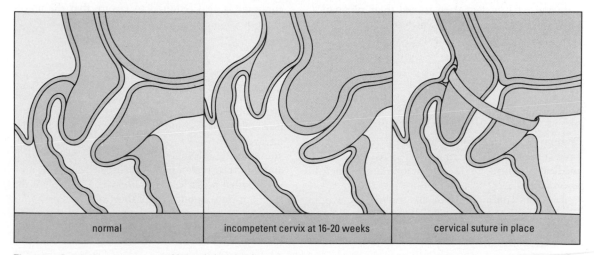

| normal | incompetent cervix at 16-20 weeks | cervical suture in place |

Fig. 5.6 Cervical incompetence. Normal view (left). Incompetent cervix at 16-20 weeks (middle). Cervical suture in place (right).

The largest group of recurrent aborters are idiopathic, i.e. no cause is found. Even after three miscarriages, at least 65 per cent of patients will carry the next pregnancy to term. If no cause is identified, it is most important to give these patients support by reassurance and regular review. Many substances have been given to these women, including vitamin C, progesterone, and HCG, but they have not been critically reviewed in double-blind controlled studies.

Induced abortion

This may be done legally in many countries within the terms of an Abortion Act, or may be carried out illegally. It may occasionally occur as a side effect of a diagnostic procedure such as chorionic villous biopsy sampling or amniocentesis.

Illegal abortions

Despite readily available contraceptive advice, there are still a large number of unwanted pregnancies each year and unfortunately this number continues to rise. The introduction of the 1967 Abortion Act in Great Britain made legal terminations more commonly available; however, the number of illegal abortions performed each year is unclear and it may be that many of those who arrive as a threatened abortion have in fact tried to end their pregnancy. However, in all countries in which an Abortion Act is introduced there is a marked reduction in the number of septic abortions admitted to hospital.

Legal termination of pregnancy

Within the terms of the Abortion Act of 1967, a pregnancy may be terminated if two registered medical practitioners are of the opinion formed in good faith that:

(i) The continuance of the pregnancy would involve a risk to the life of the pregnant woman greater than if the pregnancy was terminated.

(ii) The continuance of the pregnancy would involve risk to the physical and mental health of the pregnant woman greater than if the pregnancy was terminated.

(iii) The continuance of the pregnancy would involve risk to the physical or mental health of the existing child(ren) of the family of the pregnant woman greater than if the pregnancy was terminated.

(iv) There is a substantial risk that if a child was born it would suffer from such physical or mental abnormalities as to be seriously handicapped.

Techniques

There are various techniques employed depending on the stage of gestation and these are conveniently classified as up to twelve weeks and beyond twelve weeks.

Dilatation and curettage

Up to twelve weeks, the products of conception may be removed piecemeal from the uterus.

Suction curettage

Again up to twelve weeks, the cervix can be dilated and a suction curette inserted to empty the contents of the uterus as illustrated in Fig. 5.7. Blood loss is usually less than by curettage, but confirmatory curettage is also required to ensure that the uterus is empty.

Prostaglandins

These are used after twelve weeks and preferably after fourteen weeks. Commonly used agents are prostaglandins E_2 and $F_{2\alpha}$, which are used either intravenously, extra-amniotically or intra-amniotically. Most commonly in the UK, extra-amniotic prostaglandin E_2 is used. There are now also vaginal pessaries available which can soften the cervix or cause spontaneous abortion to occur.

Abdominal hysterotomy

This is like a miniature caesarean section with all the

attendant risks of a uterine scar. It is rarely performed nowadays.

Intra-amniotic injection

Hypertonic solutions can be injected into the amniotic sac to induce abortion. This technique is now used very infrequently because of the risk of infection.

Hysterectomy

This is only performed if there is associated obvious uterine pathology such as carcinoma of the cervix.

Complications

The main complications of termination are haemorrhage, either primary or secondary, infection, and uterine perforation (Fig. 5.8). Infection can give rise to secondary infertility and all patients should be warned of this risk. There is significant rise in the risk of subsequent spontaneous abortion following vaginal termination which may be due to traumatic cervical incompetence. Contraceptive advice is essential following termination of pregnancy.

EXTRAUTERINE PREGNANCY

An ectopic pregnancy is defined as the implantation of pregnancy outside the uterine cavity. The sites of implantation are (in order of frequency):

   (i)   Fallopian tube
   (ii) Abdominal cavity
   (iii) Ovary
   (iv) Cervix

The sites are illustrated in Fig. 5.9. Ninety-five per cent of ectopic pregnancies occur in the Fallopian tubes. The incidence is approximately one in 250 pregnancies in the UK, but can be as high as one in 30 pregnancies, particularly in the West Indies.

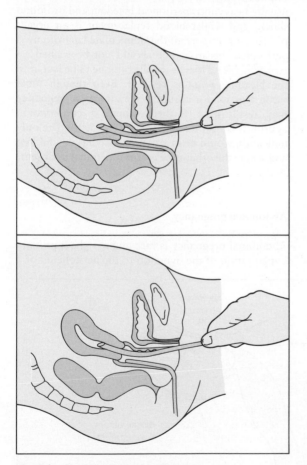

Fig. 5.7 Suction termination of pregnancy.

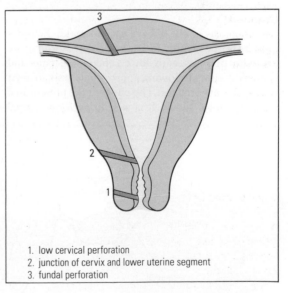

1. low cervical perforation
2. junction of cervix and lower uterine segment
3. fundal perforation

Fig. 5.8 Possible sites of uterine perforation at abortion. 1, low cervical perforation with laceration of descending branches of uterine artery; 2, perforation at junction of cervix and lower uterine segment; 3, fundal perforation.

Tubal pregnancy

The cause of tubal pregnancy is a delay in the transfer of the ovum along the Fallopian tube, due to various reasons, so that the ovum develops to the implantation stage within the tube and attaches to the endosalpinx. The tube may be congenitally abnormal, such as a diverticular tube or a long convoluted tube, or it may be distorted due to adhesions following pelvic peritionitis, often resulting from a neglected appendicitis. Chronic salpingitis causes loss of ciliary action as well as tubal occlusion. Stricture following tubal surgery may also predispose to trauma. The distal ampullary region is the most common site of implantation. If implantation occurs in the interstitial portion of the Fallopian tube, then rupture is often delayed until 16-20 weeks. The tubal epithelium tends to undergo decidua-like changes, but only to a limited extent. The trophoblast erodes into the tubal wall and eventually the gestation sac ruptures either into the lumen of the tube, causing a tubal abortion, or through the tube itself with bleeding either into the peritoneal cavity or between the folds of the broad ligament, depending on the site of the rupture.

Diagnosis

The diagnosis is not always easy to make. Ectopics must be borne in mind in any woman of reproductive age who presents with lower abdominal pain and vaginal bleeding following approximately six to eight weeks of amenorrhoea. The patient may present in a state of clinical shock. It is wise to perform vaginal examinations in such patients *only* in hospital because of the risk of rupturing an ectopic.

Common differential diagnoses include torsion of an ovarian cyst, appendicitis, haemorrhage from a ruptured follicle or salpingitis. The diagnostic test to perform, if there is doubt, is laparoscopy when the tubes can actually be visualized. Pregnancy tests, especially using beta-HCG specific tests, are often, but not always, positive, and ultrasound scan is often inconclusive.

Management

Once the diagnosis has been made, laparotomy is performed. Prior to rupture it is easy to perform a salpingectomy. If rupture has occurred there is usually heavy intraperitoneal bleeding and profound shock, and whilst blood replacement is an urgent priority, it is important that immediate laparotomy is performed, because time should not be wasted on replacing blood loss as it will continue to be lost until the bleeding point is secured. Even though tubal reconstruction for unruptured midportion pregnancy may result in a further ectopic, a conservation approach is followed by some. (Fig. 5.10). The only indication would be in a patient who has no children and where the other tube is non-functional or absent.

Abdominal pregnancy

Abdominal pregnancy is rare and may be a primary implantation of the ovum on to the peritoneum or a

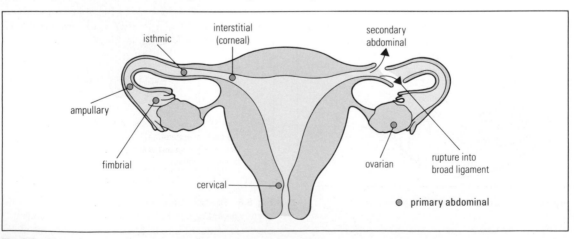

Fig. 5.9   Sites of ectopic pregnancy.

secondary implantation following tubal rupture. It is often difficult to diagnose and resembles a normal pregnancy. The fetus is easily palpable but ultrasound scans show bizarre appearances. These patients often present as acute abdominal emergencies in the second trimester. The ultrasound scan frequently shows oligohydramnios with no clear uterine outline and this is the most important diagnostic test available. It may even be possible to see the uterus as a separate entity.

Laparotomy is performed to deliver the fetus. It may be malformed due to pressure. It may not be possible or advisable to remove the placenta because it is likely to be fixed to abdominal organs so the cord is ligated and it is therefore left to be reabsorbed. Amenorrhoea may then occur for up to two years while the placenta is slowly absorbed.

Ovarian pregnancy

Fertilization of an ovum in its follicle is thought to be the cause. Rupture occurs early and the picture resembles that of a ruptured tubal pregnancy. The treatment is by oophorectomy.

Cervical pregnancy

Cervical pregnancy follows the very low implantation of a fertilized ovum. The enlarging gestation sac distends the cervix which may cause expulsive contractions. Rupture occurs into the cervical canal, the broad ligament or the vagina with consequent abortion. Cervical pregnancies are very rare and may occur without a diagnosis being made.

TROPHOBLASTIC TUMOURS

This condition results from abnormal growth of the placenta (trophoblast). Trophoblastic differentiation varies from benign hyperplasia (hydatidiform mole) to undifferentiated, highly malignant (choriocarcinoma). A precise classification is difficult, but a scheme is shown in Fig. 5.11. Even histological appearances are difficult to interpret because the usual indication of malignancy, namely invasion, is a normal feature of trophoblastic action.

Hydatiform mole

This is a vesicular degeneration of the chorionic villi and is the commonest and most benign change. They have an incidence of approximately one in 2000 pregnancies in Western countries, one in 200 in some Asian countries and one in 100 among Chinese races. Having had a hydatidiform mole, the patient has a four to five times increased incidence of another, although they are commonest in primigravidae.

Clinical manifestations
Bleeding in early pregnancy after eight weeks' amenorrhoea is common and tends to be recurrent rather than profuse. The uterus continues to grow, often appearing large for dates. The patient may present with hyperemesis, and associated hypertension and albuminuria are common. Pre-eclampsia can occur before 24 weeks in hydatidiform mole pregnancies. Cystic enlargement of the ovaries is common the result of excessive stimulation of HCG which is secreted by the molar tissue.

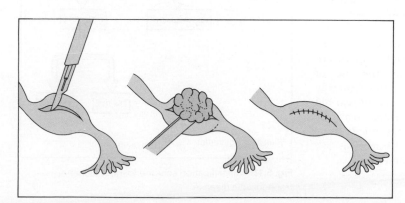

Fig. 5.10 Conservative management of unruptured midsegment tubal pregnancy. A linear incision is made along the antimesenteric border and is carried slightly beyond the area of dilatation. The ovisac and placenta are displaced from their attachments to the tubal mucosa, and the incision is closed primarily or by secondary intent.

Diagnosis

Because hydatidiform tissue produces excessive HCG, the pregnancy test is often positive even in the maximal dilutions. There is no absolute diagnostic range. Ultrasound scan usually shows a typical snowstorm appearance, often without a fetal complex at all, although with partial moles a fetal pole may be seen. Occasionally the passage of vesicles per vagina is seen. The appearance of a hydatidiform mole is shown in Fig. 5.12.

Treatment

Uterine evacuation is indicated if it has not occurred spontaneously. This can be achieved by oxytocin infusion, prostaglandins, curettage, vacuum aspiration or hysterotomy. The most commonly used method nowadays is vacuum aspiration in conjunction with oxytocin infusion. Prolonged follow-up is required as approximately 5-10 per cent of patients will progress to frank choriocarcinoma.

Prognosis

The immediate prognosis is excellent, although at one time death from haemorrhage or sepsis was approximately 10 per cent. The remote prognosis is now much more important. It hinges on the incidence of subsequent malignancies. Any type of mole may metastasise to the lungs, and pulmonary metastases may show obvious malignancy, even though the primary mole may have seemed completely benign on histological study. Two main types of gestational trophoblastic neoplasia are recognized: non-metastic disease and metastatic disease. The differentiation between the two is far from easy. More than 90 per cent will make a complete recovery and those who do recover appear to be normally fertile.

Hydatidiform mole is a premalignant lesion. The argument on how best to classify moles in terms of risk has been made obsolete by the use of chemotherapy and the decision regarding therapy rests with the clinician. For example, in a 40-year-old patient, hysterectomy would be preferable to a 1 per cent risk of choriocarcinoma, whereas in a 20-year-old woman with no children, the 10 per cent risk would probably be better than a hysterectomy.

Management

Following evacuation of the mole, the patient should be followed up after two weeks. If she has had any abnormal or excessive bleeding, then a repeat dilatation and curettage should be performed. Weekly urine assays of HCG are taken and in the majority of women, the level will have fallen to normal levels in eight to ten weeks. Persistent high titres indicate living trophoblast either within the uterus or elsewhere, in which case a repeat evacuation is indicated. Patients should be referred to recognized centres for treatment of trophoblastic diseases. Follow up includes a chest X-ray and appropriate vaginal examination at regular intervals. Urine assays start at one week, continue weekly for eight weeks and if they show an appropriate fall, monthly thereafter for up to two years.

Contraceptive advice is given, barrier methods being the most appropriate. The patient should avoid conception for at least six months and preferably for 12-24 months. If the HCG levels fail to fall, chemotherapy may be indicated.

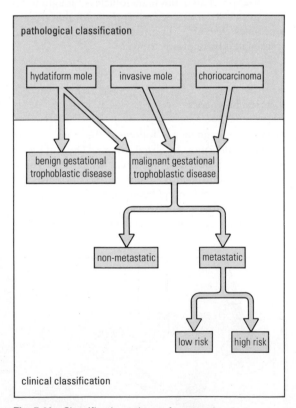

Fig. 5.11 Classification scheme for gestational trophoblastic disease.

Choriocarcinoma

This rare malignant tumour of trophoblastic tissue is, in part, paternal in origin and responds to chemotherapy better than almost any other malignant tumour. The incidence is shown in Fig. 5.12. Non-metastatic trophoblastic disease is where there is no spread outside the uterus. Metastatic spread is by direct invasion, and perforation of the uterus may occur. Blood vessels are invaded and blood transfer is the main cause of metastases, particularly to the liver, lung and brain.

Symptoms

Vaginal bleeding, particularly following hydatidiform mole, is common. Metastases may produce haemoptysis or cause obstruction of the pulmonary arterioles, producing pulmonary hypertension and congestive cardiac failure. The signs include a persistently high HCG level and an enlarged soft uterus. Chest X-ray may indicate pulmonary metastases.

Treatment

The introduction of methotrexate led to a vast improvement in the management of malignant trophoblastic disease. For best results all patients are treated in special centres. Several chemotherapeutic agents are now used, but in particular methotrexate is used in combination with other agents, depending on whether the patient is defined as low, medium or high risk.

Chemotherapy is obviously the method of choice in patients wishing to maintain childbearing capacity, but in older women a hysterectomy followed by chemotherapy is the usual regime. Irradiation can be used if metastases are resistant to drugs. Solitary lung metastases can be removed surgically.

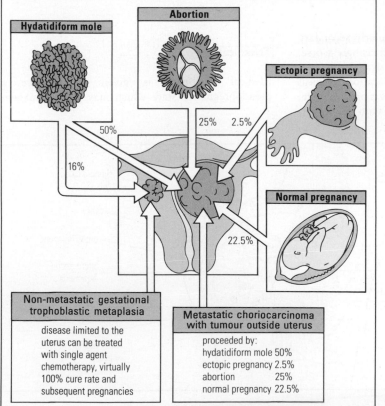

Fig. 5.12 Schematic representation of the relation of various types of pregnancy to choriocarcinoma destruens (invasive mole) and choriocarcinoma. The tendency of any one type of pregnancy to become malignant is indicated by the approximate percentages on the interconnecting lines.

85

ENDOMETRIOSIS

Endometriosis is the presence of endometrial tissue in sites other than the uterine cavity. External endometrial deposits occur in a variety of sites, particularly the ovaries, pouch of Douglas, and uterosacral ligaments, but can be found in the bowel, vagina or more distant sites such as blood vessels as shown in Fig. 5.13. Internal endometriosis or adenomyosis is confined to the myometrium and this diagnosis can only be made histologically following hysterectomy. There are various theories of aetiology including:

(i) Implantation: retrograde menstruation along the tubes can cause seedlings in the peritoneal cavity.
(ii) Venous spread which may explain distant foci.
(iii) Lymphatic spread, although this is unlikely.
(iv) Coelomic metaplasia of an embryological origin.

Symptoms

The main symptom is pain, particularly secondary dysmenorrhoea which becomes increasingly worse. The patients also complain of deep dyspareunia and sometimes pain or bleeding on defaecation. Surgical scars may be painful if endometriosis is present there. There is a definite association with infertility, although the cause is not clear as the tubes are usually patent. It could be that there is distortion or restriction of the Fallopian tube. Periods are often heavy and irregular.

Signs

Physical signs may include a fixed retroverted uterus, nodules or tenderness in the pouch of Douglas or uterosacral ligaments, and a firm or tender, enlarged ovary. Occasionally visible foci situated on the vagina or cervix may be seen as blue-black spots. The main differential diagnosis is from chronic pelvic inflammatory disease.

Diagnosis

Endometriosis is often suspected after a careful history is taken. Laparoscopy allows the diagnosis to be made and the sites identified.

Treatment

Medical treatment is given to produce a pseudopregnancy state which may give permanent

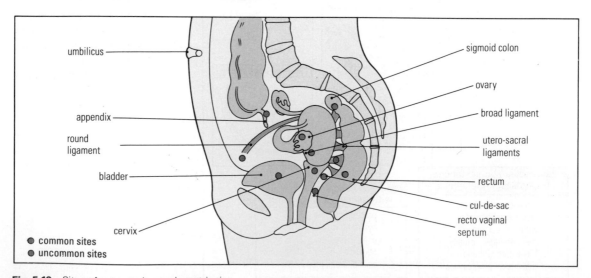

umbilicus

appendix

round
ligament

bladder

cervix

sigmoid colon

ovary

broad ligament

utero-sacral
ligaments

rectum

cul-de-sac
recto vaginal
septum

● common sites
● uncommon sites

Fig. 5.13 Sites of extrauterine endometriosis.

relief by decidualizing the ectopic endometrium which is then absorbed. The combined oral contraceptive pill may be given continuously, or Danazol, an anti-gonadotrophin, is commonly used. Treatment should be given for at least six months.

Surgery should be very conservative in those patients wishing further pregnancies. Unfortunately, pregnancy occurs in less than 30 per cent of patients and conservative surgery often gives only incomplete, temporary relief of symptoms. In particular, large ovarian cysts may need removal. Radical surgery usually consists of removal of the uterus and ovaries. There is often no point in doing only a hysterectomy, as the ovaries are a common site of endometriosis. Additional surgery may be required if other areas, such as the bowel, are involved.

ADENOMYOSIS

This occurs in slightly older patients than endometriosis. The patients are often over 35, multiparous and they often present with menorrhagia. The uterus is usually symmetrically enlarged on the examination but rarely exceeds 12 weeks in size. The treatment of choice is hysterectomy, as attempts at local incision have been unsuccessful. The diagnosis is confirmed histologically.

INFERTILITY

This is the involuntary failure to conceive within 12 months of commencing unprotected intercourse. Primary infertility is where no previous pregnancy has occured, and secondary infertility follows a previous pregnancy, whatever the outcome. About 15 per cent of couples are infertile. The source of the problem is shown in (Fig. 5.14).

Causes

Male
Failure to produce sperm in adequate numbers because of:
(i)   poor development of testes or decreasing function due to conditions such as cirrhosis of the liver;

(ii)   undescended testes;
(iii)   mumps orchiditis after 14 years of age;
(iv)   irradiation or cytotoxic therapy;
(v)   exposure to heat, such as hot baths or tight underwear;
(vi)   disease of the testes, e.g. tumours or syphilis.

Bilateral obstruction of the epididymis, vas deferens or ejaculatory ducts:
(i)   accident or operation, e.g. hernia as a child;
(ii)   infection, e.g. gonorrhoea;
(iii)   absent or gross hypoplasia. Two per cent of the population have congenital unilateral absence of the vas.

Failure to deposit sperm in the vagina, because of:
(i)   impotence;
(ii)   premature ejaculation;
(iii)   abnormality of the penis; e.g. hypospadias;
(iv)   retrograde ejaculation.

Female
Developmental. Absence of the uterus obviously causes infertility. The absence of other organs may be bypassed by new techniques.

Failure to ovulate. This may be every month or intermittent, particularly in those who have irregular cycles.

Tubal obstruction. This may result from previous salpingitis or appendicitis causing pelvic adhesions and may be partial or complete.

Endometrial disease such as tuberculous endometritis, now uncommon in the UK.

Cervical factors. Cervical mucus may be hostile to sperm, either by not allowing it to penetrate or by having antibodies to the sperm. The evaluation of the sperm and the cervical mucus is shown in Fig. 5.15. The cervix may also be distorted, either congenitally or due to previous surgery.

Tumours. Fibroids may prevent implantation of the fertilized ovum.

Relative infertility is associated with *increasing age*, particularly after age 35. After childbirth, lactation often delays ovulation and therefore may delay conception.

Investigation of infertility

A careful history must be taken from each partner. It is important to know how long the couple have been trying to conceive and whether either has previously conceived.

Contraceptive use should be noted and a careful menstrual history taken from the woman. Coital history includes frequency, dyspareunia or any premature ejaculation problems. The frequency and timing of coitus is important and the most fertile time is round about ovulation which usually occurs on the 14th day of a 28-day cycle. Coital frequency of two to three times a week is average, and all too often infrequency can be the cause of infertility. Both patients should be carefully examined, observing secondary sexual characteristics, stigmata of endocrine disease, previous operation scars, etc.

Routine investigation in the male

This includes semen analysis. This should be performed after a three-day abstinence from intercourse. Normal values are a volume of 2 to 6 ml, a density of 20-250,000,000 sperm, a motility of greater than 60 per cent, and morphology of greater than 60 per cent normal. There is wide variation of sperm counts in any individual. There should be no hesitation in repeating analysis if any of the parameters are abnormal. A summary of investigations is shown in Fig. 5.16.

Routine investigation in the female

This includes assessment of ovulation and tubal patency.

Ovulation

Basal body temperature recording may be used. When a temperature rise in mid-cycle suggests that ovulation is taking place, serum progesterone approximately one week prior to expected menstruation should be greater than 35 nmol if ovulation has occurred. Endometrial biopsy at a similar time should also be able to indicate whether the endometrium is appropriate for the cycle. Serum prolactin should be assessed in case hyperprolactinaemia is present.

Tubal patency

This can be assessed either with a hysterosalpingogram using radio-opaque dye under X-ray guidance, or by laparoscopy using methylene blue dye. The latter allows direct vision of the tubes themselves as well as being useful for demonstrating patency. Fig. 5.17 summarizes the investigations.

Management

Further investigation of the male

Further management in the male is usually undertaken by a urologist with a particular interest in male infertility. Ejaculatory failure can be identified by examining urine post-coitally, when semen should be seen. Neurological causes such as diabetic neuropathy may be identifiable. Failure of organogenesis is associated with significantly

SOURCES OF INFERTILITY	
Source of problem	**Percentage**
sole cause in the female	30
sole cause in the male	30
combined cause	30
no recognizable cause	10

Fig. 5.14 Source of infertility, with approximate percentages.

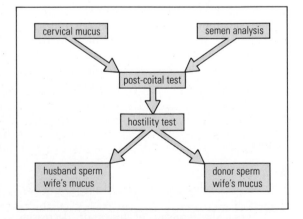

Fig. 5.15 Evaluation of cervical mucus and semen of both partners.

elevated FSH level. Unfortunately, there is little that can be done for this or many of the other causes of male infertility.

Further investigation of the female

Further investigation of the female is aimed at looking for the cause of anovulation. Treatment involves induction of ovulation as dealt with in chapter 8. If there is tubal damage, surgery may be offered. This includes:

(i) salpingolysis – the division of adhesions around the tube;

(ii) reimplantation – of the tube into the uterus;

(iii) salpingostomy – to open the blocked end of a tube.

Unfortunately, tubal surgery carries a success rate of only about 10-15 per cent. It is associated with a significantly increased risk of ectopic pregnancy.

Special techniques

Not all centres are able to offer the newer, more sophisticated techniques available for treating infertile couples. These techniques include:

(i) AIH: artificial insemination from the husband, useful where there is failure in ejaculation or intercourse is impossible.

(ii) AID: artificial insemination from donor. Care must be taken to protect the identity of the donor and ensure that both husband or wife wish this form of treatment. Inseminations are carried out twice in the periovular phase and prior investigation of female fertility is mandatory. AID is offered where the male partner has oligospermia or azospermia or carries a significant genetic risk.

(iii) GIFT: gamete intra-Fallopian tube transfer. This technique can only be used when there is normal tubal function. It is used in particular for couples with unexplained infertility. It involves the mixing together of harvested ovum and semen donated from the husband, and then reintroduction of this mixture directly into the Fallopian tube. Natural fertilization must then take place for the technique to be successful. This method is suitable for religious groups who have moral objections to the creation of an embryo outside a woman's body.

(iv) IVF: *In vitro* fertilization. This technique was originally pioneered for patients with tubal damage, although it is now used for a variety of reasons. It involves stimulation of ovarian function in the female with harvesting of the ovum. Fertilization takes place outside the body with reimplantation of the embryo, usually at the 16-cell stage. Spare embryos may be frozen and used on future occasions. Usually two or three embryos are replaced on each occasion. Unfortunately, the risk of multiple pregnancies remains higher than normal.

Both GIFT and IVF are available on the NHS in only limited centres where strict criteria are applied to the couples, such as there being no living children and a stable union, before they can go on to the waiting list.

Results

Approximately 3 per cent of women will become pregnant before the investigations are undertaken and a further 40-50 per cent will have at least one pregnancy within the next 15 years. It is important to ensure that both partners wish infertility investigations and the subsequent treatment. Some techniques require a lot of out-patient attendance and therefore patient time, in particular IVF and GIFT. Even in the best centres, the more specialized techniques have a maximum success rate of 25-30 per cent.

Adoption

Unfortunately, the waiting lists are long and the number of babies available for adoption are decreasing as a result of the increasing legal abortion rate. Couples will only be accepted after careful counselling and are usually expected to be less than 35 years of age.

INFECTIONS OF THE GENITAL TRACT

Infections of the lower genital tract are common and varied in their site. All the common organisms on the skin of the vulva, perineum and perianal areas may be associated with infection in the presence of

89

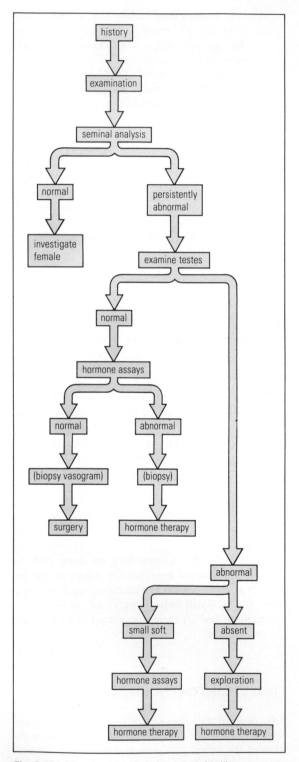

Fig. 5.16 Management of the male in infertility.

trauma to these areas or may ascend to infect the vagina or cervix. Many organisms are involved (Fig. 5.18), and many pathogens have been recognised as being transmitted sexually.

Vulvovaginitis

Following trauma, or in the presence of a foreign body, normal commensals such as streptococci can cause profuse vulvovaginitis. Rarely, infestations with amoeba, schistosomiasis or threadworms may occur.

Candida albicans (monilia or thrush organisms), trichomonas vaginalis and gardnerella are the commonest organisms found in the vagina causing abnormal discharge. All can be transmitted sexually, but are not necessarily, and they may cause little harm. Candida infections are particularly common during pregnancy and in diabetics, and following broad-spectrum antibiotic therapy. Patients usually present with irritation of the vulva and/or vagina, and discharge – white and cheesy with candida, or thin and pale green with trichomonas or gardnerella. On examination, discharge is often visible at the introitus, but will be seen on speculum examination around the cervix, and a high vaginal or endocervical swab should be taken.

Treatment is with anti-fungal agents for candida and metronidazole for trichomonas or garderella. Both partners should receive treatment simultaneously.

Superficial lesions

Superficial lesions on the vulva may be due to the following conditions:

1. Genital warts. These can be seen in the vagina, cervix, anal canal or over the perineal or perianal region. They are caused by a papilloma virus which is transmitted at coitus. They are particularly exuberant during pregnancy. Treatment is by dabbing with podophyllin resin (not in pregnancy), or diathermy. There is now evidence to suggest that the wart virus is important in the pathogenesis of CIN and carcinoma of the cervix and vagina.
2. Herpes virus type II: whilst relatively uncommon, this is a very painful condition,

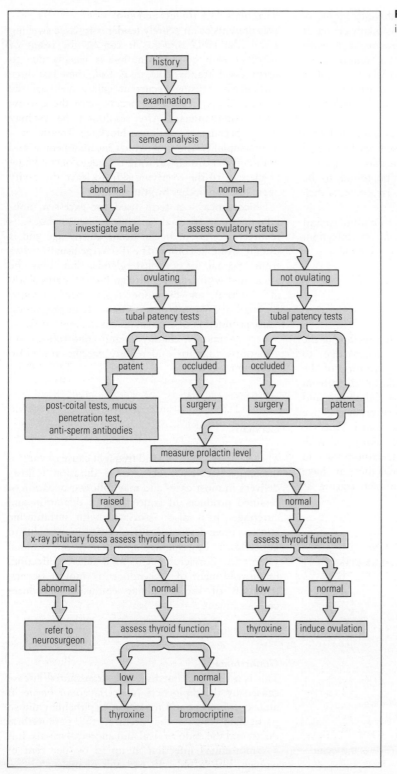

Fig. 5.17 Management of the female in infertility.

presenting with painful papulovesicular ulcers in the vulva, vagina and occasionally cervix. It is sexually transmitted. Treatment is with antivirals such as Acyclovir ointment or tablets, but is usually unsatisfactory unless commenced very early. The disease tends to recur and cannot ever be regarded as completely cured.

3. Primary syphilis presents as an indurated, firm and painless ulcer with raised borders called chancre. It can present on the vulva, vagina or cervix. Groin nodes may be found to be enlarged, firm and painless. Treatment is with penicillin.

4. Chancroid is characterized by painful genital ulcers due to *Haemophilus ducreyi* infection. Good hygiene and the use of condoms is advised.

Gonorrhoea

Gonorrhoea may present with painful swelling of the vulva, dysuria and urinary frequency due to urethritis, green vaginal discharge, irritation of the vagina, or salpingitis. Swabs should be taken from potentially infected sites including the throat and rectum and gram staining will reveal gram negative intracellular diplococci. Treatment is with Procaine penicillin 2.4 – 4.8 mU intramuscularly, or with probenecid, erythromycin or spectinomycin in patients who are allergic to penicillin or have penicillin-resistant organisms. Contact tracing is essential.

ORGANISMS INVOLVED IN LOWER GENITAL TRACT INFECTIONS

Candida albicans (thrush)
Trichomonas vaginalis
Gardnerella vaginalis
chlamydia
papilloma virus (warts)
herpes genitalis
cytomegalovirus
Neisseria gonorrhoeae (gonorrhoea)
Treponema pallidum (syphilis)

Fig. 5.18 Organisms involved in infections of the lower genital tract.

Bartholins duct abscess and cyst

This presents as an acutely tender soft tissue swelling within the labia minora. It can be the result of infection with gonorrhoea, but is usually due to streptococci, staphyococci, or *E. Coli*, these last three particularly causing recurrent enlargement of the glands. Abcess formation occurs once the narrow duct becomes infected. After resolution, the cyst may remain because of continued blockage. Treatment is to marsupialize the cyst which means opening and draining it and then suturing the edges of the lining of the cyst to the overlying skin to leave the cavity open. Healing occurs by granulation.

Leucorrhoea – a term used for excessive non-inflammatory vaginal discharge, leucorrhoea is relatively common. It can occur at any age and is usually white in colour. The discharge usually arises from vaginal or cervical glands, but may be associated with trauma, foreign bodies (particularly in children), or hormone replacement therapy. Elevated oestrogen levels, particularly in pregnancy, cause production of cervical mucus in large amounts.

Less commonly, chlamydia and gonorrohoea can also cause vaginitis and require specific antibiotic treatment.

Cervicitis

This is a very common and frequent cause of vaginal discharge. Cervicitis of variable duration follows delivery in most cases and may follow evacuation of retained products of conception or dilatation and curettage. It is also associated with intrauterine contraceptive devices. Acute cervicitis may be due to gonorrhoea or chlamydia, often with minimal symptoms. Cervicitis begins as a surface infection, but involvement of the endocervix rapidly occurs. Irritation of the glandular epithelium produces copious mucus.

Gonorrhoea

This is a legally defined sexually transmitted disease caused by the diplococci *Neisseria gonorrhoeae*. It attacks columnar and transitional epithelium and so particulary affects the urethra, the paraurethral ducts, and the endocervical and anorectal canals. It is a symptomless infection in up to 60 per cent of women, but in only 10 per cent of males.

Syphilis

This is one of the more reliably reported sexually transmitted diseases, although the incidence varies In the UK, as in many other countries, pregnant women are routinely screened for syphilis.

Chlamydia

Chlamydia trachomatis is an intracellular sexually transmitted bacterial pathogen and is now the leading cause of acute pelvic inflammatory disease. It is more prevalent than gonorrhoea in many countries. It is the most commonly reported sexually transmitted organism in the genitourinary medicine clinics in this country. Between 20 and 40 per cent of sexually active women have antibodies against chlamydia, and between 10 and 30 per cent of women with acute pelvic inflammatory disease who do not have positive cultures for chlamydia have antibody titres suggestive of acute chlamydial infection.

Chlamydia infection of either the lower or upper genital tract is therefore seen most frequently in the young women who are sexually active. Clinically, chlamydia produces a mild form of salpingitis with an insidious onset. Chlamydia may remain latent in the Fallopian tubes for months following initial colonization of the upper genital tract. The correlation of the intensity of the symptoms of pelvic inflammatory disease and the state of the tubes is poor. Women with chlamydia may have minor symptoms, yet can be found to have evidence of severe inflammatory processes visible on laparoscopic examination; this is nowadays considered to be a major factor in tubal infertility.

Acquired Immune Deficiency Syndrome (AIDS)

AIDS is the clinical end-stage of human immunodeficiency virus (HIV) infection, which results in severe and/or irreversible immune suppression. After a certain amount of immune system damage has occurred, the individual becomes susceptible to many opportunistic infections and cancers. These infections and cancers are indirect markers of the acquired immunodeficiency caused by HIV.

HIV is a retrovirus which reproduces in human cells. Retroviruses have a unique way of reproducing themselves because they possess an enzyme: reverse transcriptase. As a consequence, when the host cell divides, copies of the virus are produced along with the daughter host cells, and each new cell contains the virus. So once the virus enters a host cell, permanent infection is established. The retrovirus may not, however, produce ill effects for a number of years, and the activating or initiating factors are unknown at present. HIV infection selectively infects macrophages as well as other cells of the immune system such as T-helper cells. When the virus reproduces, it reduces the number of T-helper cells and prevents surviving cells from functioning properly. The loss on immunity is selective and principally affects those parts of the immune system involved defending against parasitic, viral and fungal organisms. Thus individuals with AIDS develop unusual infections, yet are still able to resist more common illnesses.

The HIV virus has been isolated from plasma, semen, saliva, tears, CSF, urine, breast milk and cervical mucus. Of these, only blood, semen, and cervical mucus have been shown to be infective pathways. Anal intercourse is dangerous because it is traumatic to rectal mucosa, and because semen is immunosuppressive which reduces the resistance to HIV. Vaginal mucosa and cervical epitheleum are more resistant to trauma, but with either form of intercourse barrier condom contraception is protective.

Infection with HIV falls into three main groups:

(i)   The asymptomatic carrier with antibodies present.
(ii) Persistent generalised lymphadenopathy.
(iii) HIV-related disease including AIDS.

Although AIDS represents the end-stage of HIV infection, it is not known how many individuals with HIV will develop AIDS or other symptoms. There is, at present, no cure for AIDS and once established, death occurs within 18 to 24 months. HIV infection can be transmitted to the fetus during pregnancy or to the baby at delivery. The risk of intrauterine infection for the fetus of an HIV-positive mother is estimated to be 25-50 per cent. There is uncertainty whether pregnancy increases the incidence of AIDS in HIV-positive mothers, but there are some reports that it does.

Because AIDS cannot be treated, screening for HIV is not acceptable, and consent and counselling are therefore required before testing for HIV antibody.

There are inevitable ethical and legal problems if a test proves to be positive, so women at a high risk of exposure to the virus can only be encouraged to volunteer to be tested. It must also be appreciated that detectable antibodies to HIV may not develop for several months after exposure and so a repeat test may be required. Whenever a woman requests a test or is encouraged to have a test for HIV antibody, she must have full details of the medical, psychological, legal, and social implications of a positive finding.

Risk of infection for those dealing with patients, infected or not, have been greatly exaggerated and the risk of contacting hepatitis is far greater. Non-sexual contact between HIV-positive individuals and those working in the hospital environment carries no risk. The standard precaution when handling a blood sample will avoid any risk. The same techniques that are used to avoid contact with Hepatitis B virus should be used for HIV. It must be remembered that at present the syndrome of AIDS is seen only in a small proportion of those infected with HIV.

Infections of the upper genital tract

Pelvic inflammatory disease (Fig. 5.19) is defined as an acute febrile illness in a woman with pelvic pain and vaginal discharge. It is otherwise called acute salpingitis, although the endometrium may also be infected. It is a common cause of admission to hospital, particularly in young women. Most cases are due to bacterial infections caused be streptococci, staphylococci, chlamydia or gonorrhoea. Rare infections include actinomycosis and schistosomiasis. Causes of infection of the upper genital tract are shown in Fig. 5.20.

Epidemiology
Seventy per cent of women with salpingitis are 25 years old or younger; 30 per cent have their babies before the age of 20; and 75 per cent are multiparous. There are approximately 250 000 000 new cases of gonorrhoea each year worldwide. The increased incidence and prevalence of pelvic infection is felt to be due to the more urbanised population with early and more promiscuous sexual activity. It does not appear to have been greatly influenced by the knowledge of the risks of AIDS (HIV infection).

Bacteriology
An acute pyogenic infection may develop into a chronic hydrosalpinx or tubo-ovarian abscess (Fig. 5.21). Gonorrhoea frequently causes peritonitis once acute salpingitis is established. A tubo-ovarian abscess may result. Gonorrhoea rarely infects the tubes after the first occasion, but flare-ups occur due to secondary invaders. The chlamydial organism accounts for half of the cases of pelvic inflammatory disease in women under 25 years of age and is a frequent cause of tubal damage, which is out of proportion to the clinical severity of the disease. The Fitz-Hugh-Curtis syndrome is an unusual complication when perihepatitis occurs secondary to pelvic infection. Treatment is with tetracycline or erythromycin.

Sequelae
Infertility occurs in approximately 20 per cent of cases after pelvic infection. Chronic infection results in chronic pelvic pain and dyspareunia and often heavy, irregular menstruation. The risk of ectopic pregnancy is increased due to tubal damage.

Clinical features
Most patients present with a combination of the following:-
  (i)   Acute pelvic pain.
  (ii) Pyrexia, with a high intermittent fever up to 40°C.
  (iii) Tender adnexae, or possibly unilateral or bilateral swellings.
  (iv) Raised white cell count and ESR.
  (v)   Menstrual irregularities: salpingitis may be exacerbated by menstruation.

Diagnosis
Swabs are taken for organisms, including endocervical swabs in special medium for chlamydia. Blood may also be taken for chlamydia titres and a white cell count. Direct microscopy of the discharge is often quicker and many organisms may be identified. Most patients are treated on clinical grounds, but laparoscopy is the most reliable diagnostic measure. At laparoscopy, findings are likely to be oedema and swelling of the Fallopian

tubes, erythema of the tubes, and a seropurulent exudate on the tube and its fimbrial end.

Treatment

Antibiotic therapy is commenced once all the swabs have been taken. If specific organisms are identified or grown, then treatment should obviously reflect these. Often no results are available and broad-spectrum treatment is given to cover the likely organisms. Ampicillin, erythromycin, or cephalosporins are used, along with metronidazole (Flagyl) which covers the anaerobic organisms. Tetracyclines may also be used, as long as

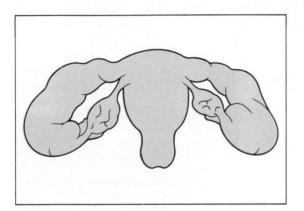

Fig. 5.19 Gross appearance in pelvic inflammatory disease.

UPPER GENITAL TRACT CAUSES OF INFECTION OF
sexually transmitted diseases, e.g. chlamydia and gonorrhoea.
post-delivery or miscarriage
surgical procedure, e.g. D & C, insertion of coil, or hysterosalpingogram
direct ascending spread of infection (often anaerobic) from vagina to cervix
secondary infection from an inflamed cervix or in association with other disease such as schistosomiasis or tubo-ovarian abscess

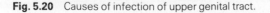

Fig. 5.20 Causes of infection of upper genital tract.

pregnancy is excluded, as they are very effective for treating chlamydia. If there is a possibility the patient may be pregnant, erythromycin is used instead.

Surgical drainage of the pyosalpinx may be required, but this is unusual. Abdominal surgery is contraindicated in acute conditions. In chronic salpingitis, pelvic clearance may be the best alternative to relieve pain and menstrual irregularities. Unfortunately, the uterus may become fixed in retroversion and cause dyspareunia. If fixed, there is little treatment to offer apart from a pelvic clearance. Tubal surgery following pelvic infection has very poor results (Fig. 5.22).

Pelvic tuberculosis

This has shown a massive decline since the introduction of antituberculous antibiotics. Sadly, the prospect of successful pregnancy after treatment remains extremely low and the incidence of ectopic pregnancy high. Tuberculous peritonitis can occur in the indigenous population, though it is more common in immigrants.

BENIGN LESIONS OF THE GENITAL TRACT

Vulva and vagina

Dermatological conditions can affect the vulva and include eczema, or psoriasis. The vulval dystrophies include a number of disorders associated with abnormal and disorderly epithelial activity which can be premalignant. Some are simply due to senile atrophy.
Swellings include:
(i) Haematoma due to trauma.
(ii) Infective causes such as infected hair follicles.
(iii) A prolapse such as cystocele or rectocele.
(iv) Cysts, such as sebaceous, inclusion dermoid, Wolffian duct remnant and endometriosis.
(v) Varicocities of the vulva.
(vi) Enlargement of the Bartholin gland. This is usually due to an infection which can cause an abscess. After an infection has occurred, the main duct of the gland becomes blocked and a Bartholin's cyst may form.
  Marsupialization rather than excision is considered to be the best management.

95

(vii) Urethral and para-urethral conditions such as a caruncle.

(viii)Inguinal hernias or hydroceles of the canal of Nook.

(ix) Benign neoplasms such as papillomas, fibromas, lipomas or hidradenomas.

The simplest measures should be taken to treat all these conditions.

Cervix

Cervical erosions

An erosion or ectopy is the replacement of normal squamous epithelium on the vaginal aspect of the cervix by columnar epithelium (which normally lines the endocervix). It is very common in women of reproductive age, particularly those using the oral

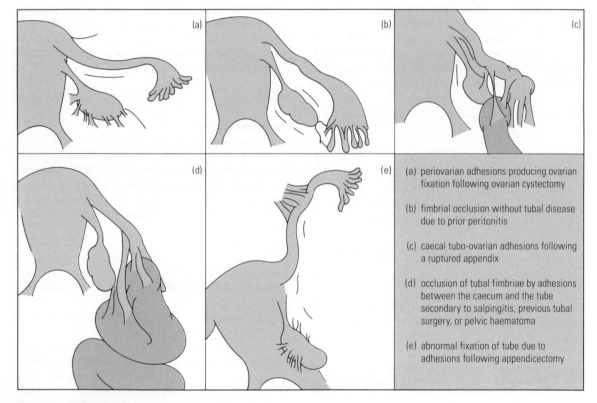

(a) periovarian adhesions producing ovarian fixation following ovarian cystectomy

(b) fimbrial occlusion without tubal disease due to prior peritonitis

(c) caecal tubo-ovarian adhesions following a ruptured appendix

(d) occlusion of tubal fimbriae by adhesions between the caecum and the tube secondary to salpingitis, previous tubal surgery, or pelvic haematoma

(e) abnormal fixation of tube due to adhesions following appendicectomy

Fig. 5.21 Tubo-ovarian distortion produced by adhesions.

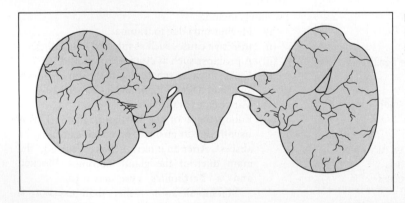

Fig. 5.22 Bilateral 'retort'-shaped Fallopian tubes due to chronic salpingitis.

contraceptive pill. Symptoms tend to be limited to mucoid, mucopurulent discharge, and occasional postcoital bleeding, although many patients are asymptomatic. If the symptoms are troublesome, then the erosion may be treated by cautery or diathermy, but unfortunately they frequently recur. Different cervical lesions are illustrated in Fig. 5.23.

Cervical polyps

These are common and are small, pedunculated and often sessile. They can occur at any time after the menarche and are usually asymptomatic. They may cause intermenstrual or postcoital bleeding and should be removed as polyps are potential focus of cancer. Methods of removing a cervical polyp are shown in Fig. 5.24.

Cervical intraepithelial neoplasia (CIN)

CIN forms a continual process which begins with mild dysplasia and ends with invasive carcinoma (Fig. 5.25). It usually arises within the transformation zone. The site from which abnormal cells arise may be detected by the application of acetic acid or Schiller's iodine in which the non-staining (glycogen-free) area indicates where biopsies should be taken. The degree of CIN is determined by the extent to which the neoplastic cells have involved the full thickness of cervical epithelium. It is classified as mild, moderate or severe dysplasia, or CIN I, CIN II or CIN III respectively. Carcinoma *in situ* is where the full thickness of the epithelium is composed of undifferentiated neoplastic cells. It is important to identify the degree of abnormality, both of the cervix and, if appropriate, of the vagina (where similar changes can occur) to provide appropriate treatment. For mild abnormalities (CIN I), follow-up with a repeat smear may be all that is necessary until a normal report is obtained. For moderate dysplasia (CIN II), treatment may involve eradication therapy such as diathermy or laser, or excision by cone biopsy; (see Gynaecological Operations). Severe dysplasia or carcinoma *in situ* (CIN III) needs at least a cone biopsy or laser cone treatment; a hysterectomy is sometimes appropriate. The progression of the disease must be carefully watched for some will go on to develop malignant changes if not treated early and promptly, hence the importance of regular cervical smears.

Uterus

Endometrial polyps (Fig. 5.26)

These are usually multiple, and are present before the menopause. They may be an element of endometrial hyperplasia (Fig. 5.27). Most are symptomless, but they can be associated with menorrhagia, intermenstrual bleeding, postcoital bleeding or postmenopausal bleeding. They are easily removed by dilatation and curettage.

Uterine Fibroids

Fibroids are fibromuscular (leiomyomata) tumours and are the commonest tumour in the female, being present in 30 per cent of women over 35 years. They are slow growing and, although they are present much earlier, they are not often diagnosed before the age of 35 years. The patients are usually of low or no parity and endometriosis may co-exist. Fibroids are much more common in black women.

Aetiology

Aetiology is unknown, but may be related to oestrogen stimulation. Fibroids are classified according to the site of occurrence as shown in Fig. 5.28.

(i) Subserous where the fibroids project into the peritoneal surface of the uterus.
(ii) Intramural: within the uterine wall.
(iii) Submucous: these indent the uterine cavity and may be extruded through the cervix.
(iv) Cervical.

Macroscopic features

Fibroids are usually multiple, have a firm whirled cut surface and exude a capsule from which they can be enucleated. They may become very large. Fibroids may undergo various degenerative changes:

(i) Atrophy.
(ii) Hyaline degeneration is present in most moderate to large fibroids.
(iii) Cystic degeneration which often follows hyaline degeneration.
(iv) Fatty degeneration.
(v) Calcification.

(vi) Red degeneration typically occurs during pregnancy where there is usually an infarction at the centre of the fibroid during the middle of pregnancy. The patient presents with pain.

Other changes due to fibroids can include torsion, haemorrhage or infection and very rarely, malignant (sarcomatous) change in approximately 0.05 per cent of fibroids.

Symptoms

Fibroids are often asymptomatic, especially small fibroids after the menopause. Abdominal swelling may occur if the fibroids are large enough. Patients may complain of pressure effects or retention of urine. Oedema is also common. Menorrhagia occurs because of the increased bleeding area, increased vascularity, the possible associated endometrial hyperplasia and impaired uterine contractivity. Pain may occur when there is torsion of the fibroids, degeneration or sarcomatous change.

Effects of fibroids on pregnancy

Fibroids may cause infertility by tubal distortion or occlusion. Submucous fibroids may prevent implantation or cause early abortion. As pregnancy progresses fibroids may cause confusion as to uterine size. A cervical or low-lying fibroid may give rise to an unstable lie, or may obstruct labour. The presence of fibroids may interfere with normal contraction and involution of the uterus and predispose to primary postpartum haemorrhage.

The effects of pregnancy on fibroids

Because of the hormonal changes in pregnancy, the fibroids increase in size and become much softer. Fibroids which were clinically obvious at booking are often only detectable in late pregnancy. As the uterus grows the fibroids tend to be drawn up and so cause few problems. During pregnancy and the early puerperium fibroids are particularly liable to undergo red degeneration. Fibroids are then very tender and may be mistaken for a small placental abruption.

Treatment

Treatment depends on the age and parity of the patient, the size and number of fibroids, the symptoms and complications.

(i) No treatment is an option, particularly if the fibroids are small and symptomless.

(ii) Myomectomy may be performed if further pregnancy is wanted and the fibroids may interfere with fertility.

(iii) Hysterectomy is usually easier than myomectomy and has a lower morbidity. It is the treatment of choice once the family is complete.

(iv) Polypectomy: curettage or excision of the vaginal myometa for fibroid polyps.

Ovary

Benign conditions related to the ovary will be discussed in the section on ovarian tumours.

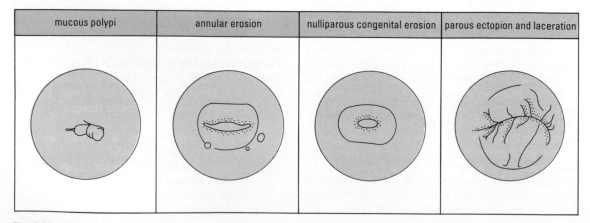

| mucous polypi | annular erosion | nulliparous congenital erosion | parous ectopion and laceration |

Fig. 5.23 Different cervical lesions.

MALIGNANT LESIONS OF THE GENITAL TRACT

Vulva

Vulval carcinoma is a disease of older women, but rarer tumours may occur at younger ages. It is the fourth most common female genital tract cancer. There is an interrelationship with neoplasias of the cervix and vagina, and approximately 15-30 per cent of women with vulval carcinoma will have had, or will develop, intraepithelial or invasive lesions of the cervix.

The types of tumour are shown in Fig. 5.29.

Symptoms and signs

An ulcer or papillary lesion may develop after a period of pruritus vulvae; continued growth is

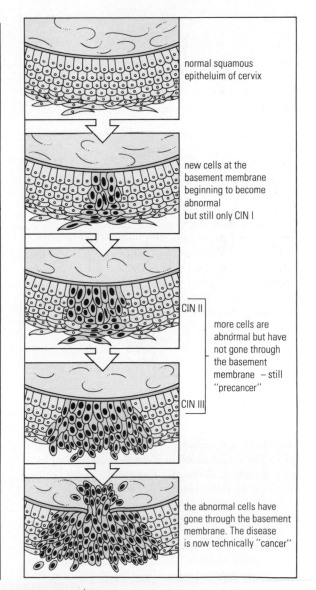

normal squamous epitheluim of cervix

new cells at the basement membrane beginning to become abnormal but still only CIN I

CIN II

more cells are abnormal but have not gone through the basement membrane – still "precancer"

CIN III

the abnormal cells have gone through the basement membrane. The disease is now technically "cancer"

Fig. 5.24 Removal of a cervical polyp by twisting (top), excision (middle) and ligating and excision (bottom).

Fig. 5.25 Progression of cervical intraepithelial neoplasia (CIN).

torsion and twisting of pedicle

excision of endocervical polyp

excision and ligation of endocervical polyp

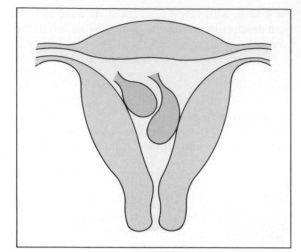

Fig. 5.26 Endometrial polyps.

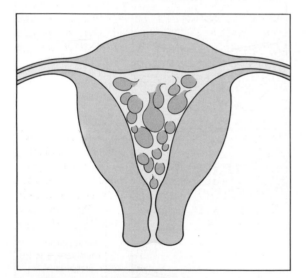

Fig. 5.27 Endometrial hyperplasia.

ultimately accompanied by bleeding, infection and pain. The major problem is the delayed presentation and therefore diagnosis. Commonly most lesions occur on the labia, clitoris or perineum.

Spread
The primary route of spread is lymphatic (Fig. 5.30), usually to the superficial and deep inguinal and femoral nodes, and then to the external iliac and obturator nodes. The common iliac and para, aortic

nodes are involved in late cases. Direct spread is into the urethra, vagina or rectum. Contralateral involvement is not uncommon.

Treatment
Surgery
Primary treatment is surgical, involving radical vulvectomy and bilateral lymphadenectomy. The major postoperative complication is wound necrosis. Patients often need a relatively long hospital stay for the wound to heal adequately.

Radiotherapy
Preoperative radiation may decrease the size of the lesion and make operation possible. Unfortunately, ulceration or fibrosis of the surrounding skin is not uncommon. It may be used for selective recurrences in patients not suitable for further surgery.

Prognosis
The overall survival rate is 60-70 per cent following complete surgical treatment. However, with nodes or metastases the five-year survival rate drops to about 30 per cent. In cases of malignant melanoma, survival to five years is very rare.

Vagina

Primary carcinoma accounts for 1-2 per cent of all gynaecological malignancies and usually develops in women over 60 years of age, although it may occur in children. Daughters of mothers who received diethylstilboestrol during early pregnancy may develop clear cell adenocarcinoma of the cervix or vagina. This is most likely to occur in women aged 10-30 years. The upper third of the vagina is the commonest site, but it may be a multicentric tumour and can involve both the vagina and cervix. Squamous carcinoma is the most common variety accounting for approximately 75 per cent of all primary vaginal carcinomas. The lymphatic spread is shown in Fig. 5.31. Secondary tumour from the cervix, endometrium or vulva are, of course, more common than primary carcinomas.

Symptoms and signs

The most common presenting complaint is painless bleeding or profuse vaginal discharge. Occasionally a vaginal mass may be noted or constipation due to pressure effects on the rectum. Pain and weight loss are manifestations. The tumour is usually ulcerative and firm to the touch.

Treatment

Radiotherapy is used for squamous carcinomas, particularly in advanced cases or where the patient is unsuitable for surgery. Surgery is used for carcinomas close to the introitus; the procedures are similar to those for vulval tumours or for radioresistant tumours such as sarcomas.

Prognosis

This depends on the type, location and extent of the tumour and the adequacy of treatment. The overall five-year survival is about 30 per cent. Five-year survival rate Stage I is approximately 85 per cent falling to 40 per cent in Stage III. There is no five-year survivors for Stage IV.

Cancer of the cervix is the commonest malignancy of the femoral reproductive tract. It is estimated that approximately 2 per cent of women aged over 40 will develop cancer of the cervix. The average age at diagnosis is 45, but in more recent years there has been a growing number of women in their early twenties or thirties presenting with a lesion.

Aetiology

The precise aetiology remains uncertain, but there are several well established associations. Cervical cancer is most common in parous women between 40 and 50 years of age. Early age at first coitus is felt to be highly significant, as is promiscuity. Papilloma virus and herpes virus have been implicated and may act as a promoting factor. The disease is far more common in the lower socioeconomic groups and thus, unfortunately those least likely to have cervical smears.

Staging for the disease is shown in Fig. 5.32 and 5.33.

Spread

This may be direct to the vagina, parametrium, body of the uterus, bladder, rectum, and pelvic wall. Lymphatic spread (Fig. 5.34) occurs in the parametrial glands, the iliac and obturator glands and then the aortic group. Blood spread is late and occurs mostly to lungs and skin.

Symptoms

These lesions are often asymptomatic until well advanced. Early symptoms include abnormal bleeding which may be slight and neglected. Vaginal discharge may be blood-stained. Super-added infection of the neoplastic tissue causes an offensive discharge. Severe haemorrhage, profuse offensive discharge and fistula formation are all late

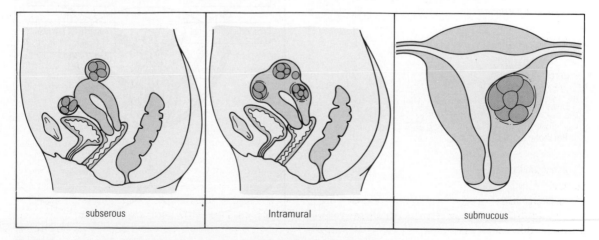

| subserous | Intramural | submucous |

Fig. 5.28 Leiomyomas (fibroids) of the uterus classified according to location.

symptoms. Bladder invasion presents as frequency, dysuria, and haematuria while bowel involvement leads to diarrhoea, rectal bleeding and possibly obstruction. Pain is a late symptom and is due to involvement of the nerve trunks of the lumbar sacral plexus or pain associated with ureteric obstruction.

Signs
In carcinoma *in situ* and microinvasive carcinoma, the cervix may appear normal. In malignant disease there may be evidence of incidental pre-existing disease. In advanced cases there will warty protrusions of the squamocolumnar junction which bleed readily and which will develop either into a papillary or exophytic-like growth, or there will be an ulcerated growth with a cauliflower-rolled friable margin. A cervical ulcer spreading into the vaginal wall or contact bleeding following a smear, is suspicious. The lesion feels hard, nodular, and craggy on palpation, and local spread can be felt.

Management
The diagnosis must be confirmed histologically by biopsy. If there is an obvious tumour present this may be confirmed by direct biopsy, but often the diagnosis is made by cone biopsy. An accurate assessment of the spread is made by vaginal and rectal examination under anaesthetic with curettage and cystoscopy. Other investigations include a chest X-ray and intravenous pyelogram. If available, nuclear magnetic resonance or a CT scan is performed to identify enlarged pelvic lymph nodes. Definitive treatment is either radiotherapy or surgery.

Radiotherapy
This is the treatment of choice for all advanced cases. It employs the intracavity insertion of a radium or caesium implant into the uterus, vaginal applicators around the cervix, and the application of megavoltage X-ray therapy to the pelvic lymph nodes. After-loading techniques are now favoured to avoid radiation exposure to those involved in treating these patients (Fig. 5.35).

Surgery
Surgery is employed in certain cases. In carcinoma *in situ*, a cone biopsy or ordinary hysterectomy suffices. Early malignant lesions, e.g. Stage I and early Stage

MALIGNANT LESIONS OF THE VULVA	
Types of malignant vulval tumour	**Percentage**
squamous carcinoma	85
melanoma	5
sarcoma	2
basal cell carcinoma	1
Bartholin's gland tumour	1
adenocarcinoma	<1
undifferentiated	<5

Fig. 5.29 Types of malignant vulval lesion.

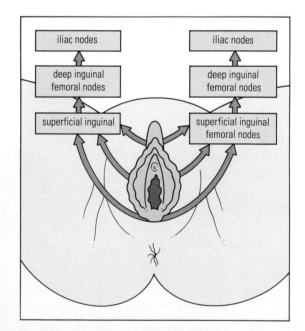

Fig. 5.30 Lymphatic drainage of the vulva.

II, may be removed surgically. The operation involves removal of the uterus, cervix, upper third of the vagina, tubes, and pelvic lymphatics. The ovaries are removed in older women, but are generally conserved in women under the age of 40. In advanced cases and some cases of recurrent disease after radiotherapy, removal of the bladder and/or rectum may be needed by procedures known as exenterations. This will involve the formation of an ileal conduit, or colostomy, or both. Surgery is the treatment of choice in young women with early lesions.

Results

The five-year survival rates are 90 per cent for Stage I, falling to 15 per cent for Stage IV. Squamous carcinoma is the most common type, accounting for 85-90 per cent, with adenosquamous or adenocarcinoma accounting for 10-15 per cent.

Uterus

Carcinoma of the endometrium of the uterus occurs in a markedly different group of women from carcinoma of the cervix. The patients tend to be older (often over 50 years of age), nulliparous and are often slightly obese, diabetic or hypertensive.

Staging of carcinoma of the uterus is shown in Fig. 5.36.

Spread

Spread may be direct into and through the uterine muscle and down to the cervix (Fig. 5.37). Late spread occurs to the Fallopian tubes, ovaries and bony pelvis. Lymphatic spread occurs to the pelvic and aortic nodes, and blood spread may occur to the ovaries and lungs.

Symptoms

The most common and often the only symptom is post-menopausal bleeding. In younger women, intermenstrual loss may occur. Vaginal discharge and pain are late symptoms. The signs are few, but uterine enlargement may be felt, particularly in postmenopausal women. Screening procedures are of limited value in this condition compared with cervical carcinoma. Diagnosis is confirmed histologically after curettage, and all women with postmenopausal bleeding must have dilatation and curettage to exclude carcinoma of the uterus.

Treatment

Treatment is primarily surgical with the removal of the uterus, ovaries, tubes and cuff of the vagina. Radiotherapy may be employed preoperatively or postoperatively to prevent further implantation of the tumour, or it may be the only method of treatment if the patient is unfit for surgery. Hormone therapy using progestogens can be employed in patients unfit for surgery or for recurrences after surgery, and it is often employed as an adjunct to surgery instead of radiotherapy. The overall five-year survival rate is approximately 70 per cent and is highest if the lesion has not penetrated the myometrium. The prognosis for carcinoma of the endometrium stage-for-stage is similar to carcinoma of the cervix, but 90 per cent of cases are Stage I carcinomas of the endometrium.

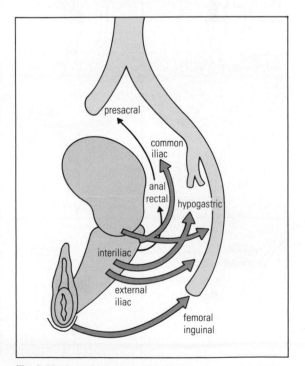

Fig. 5.31 Lymphatic drainage of the vagina.

STAGING OF CARCINOMA OF THE CERVIX	
Stage 0:	carcinoma *in situ*
Stage I:	divided into IA (microinvasive) and IB (any lesion restricted to the cervix)
Stage II:	carcinoma has spread to the vagina, but not to its lower third, and/or the lesion has spread into the parametrium, but not as far as the pelvic wall
Stage III:	carcinoma has spread to the lower third of the vagina and/or has reached the bony pelvis
Stage IV:	invasion of the rectum or bladder, or with the presence of distant metastases.

Fig. 5.32 Staging of carcinoma of the cervix.

Choriocarcinoma

Choriocarcinoma has been discussed previously (see p. 85)

Sarcoma of the uterus

This is a very rare tumour, of which three types are recognized.

(i) Endometrial stromal sarcoma.

(ii) Myometrial sarcoma, which may arise in a fibroid.

(iii) Sarcoma botryoides, which is a rare lesion seen in young girls.

Unfortunately, this rapidly involves the cervix and vagina and is almost always fatal.

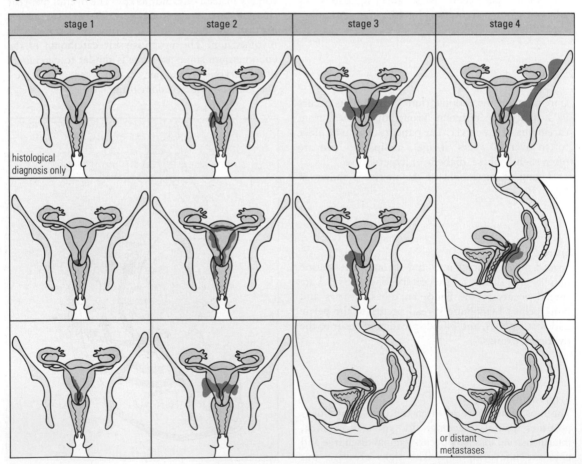

Fig. 5.33 Clinical staging of carcinoma of the cervix.

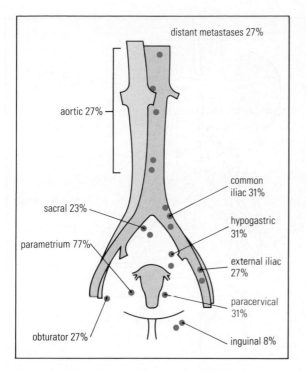

Fig. 5.34 Frequency of lymph node metastases in cervical carcinoma.

Fallopian tube

Carcinoma of the Fallopian tube is exceedingly rare, and its cause is unknown. It tends to occur in women aged 40-60 years and consists of a papillary adenocarcinoma. Patients present with a warty vaginal discharge or abdominal pain. Treatment is by total abdominal hysterectomy and bilateral salpingo-oophorectomy followed by external radiotherapy and possibly chemotherapy. The five-year survival rate is between 5 and 25 per cent, and this reflects the late diagnosis in most cases.

Ovarian Tumours

The most common ovarian tumours are benign serous tumours (25 per cent), benign mucinous tumours (25 per cent) and dermoid cysts (20 per cent). About 25 per cent of ovarian tumours are malignant, and they cause more deaths than carcinoma of the cervix (about 4000 per year in England and Wales; Fig. 5.38). Unfortunately, there is at present no satisfactory screening procedure, although regular vaginal examination seems to be

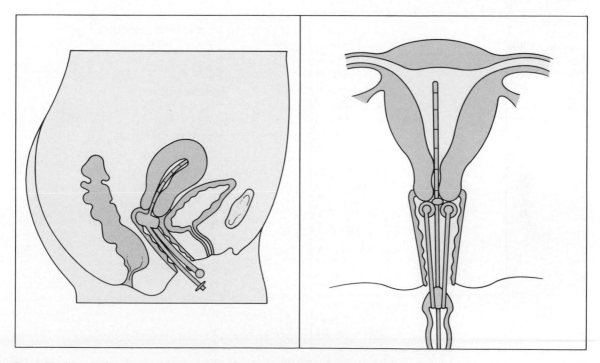

Fig. 5.35 Intrauterine caesium application for cervical cancer. using afterloading apparatus.

STAGING OF CARCINOMA OF THE UTERUS	
Stage I	carcinoma confined to the corpus
Stage II:	carcinoma involving corpus and carvix
Stage III:	carcinoma situated outside the uterus, but not outside the true pelvis
Stage IV:	carcinoma has extended into the true pelvis and may involve the mucosa of the bladder or rectum, or there are distant metastases

Fig. 5.36 Staging of carcinoma of the uterus.

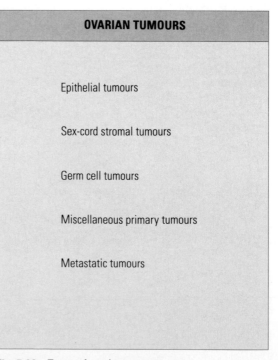

Fig. 5.37 Spread of endometrial carcinoma.

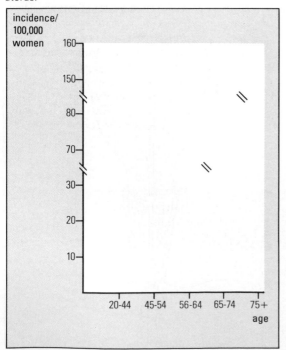

Fig. 5.38 Incidence of ovarian cancer according to age.

OVARIAN TUMOURS
Epithelial tumours
Sex-cord stromal tumours
Germ cell tumours
Miscellaneous primary tumours
Metastatic tumours

Fig. 5.39 Types of ovarian tumours.

best. Hence, bimanual examination is essential when doing cervical screening. Ultrasound scanning has some benefit, but is not readily available as a screening tool.

The main groups of ovarian tumours are shown in Fig. 5.39.

Common epithelial tumours

The commonest types of epithelial ovarian tumours are the mucinous and serous, but endometriod, mesonephroid and Brenner tumours may also occur (Fig. 5.40).

Benign mucinous cystadenoma

This is a multilocular or unilocular cyst lined by tall columnar epithelial cells similar to that of the endocervix. Microscopically there is an outer fibrous capsule, a middle layer of stroma supporting the walls of the small cysts and possible elastic tissue and smooth muscle. Complications which can occur include torsion of the cyst, secondary infection, malignant transformation and pseudomyxoma of the peritoneum – a rare occurrence consequent upon rupture of the cyst.

Benign serous cystadeoma

This is an ovarian tumour lined by epithelium which is similar to that of the Fallopian tube. Microscopic examination reveals three types: (1) cystic; (2) papillary; and (3) adenomatous. The wall is composed of an outer fibrous and inner epithelial layer with the middle made up of loose connective tissue. The epithelial lining may appear stratified because of tangential cutting of the papilla with the nuclei being at different heights, even though there is only a single layer of cells. It is sometimes difficult to decide whether a cyst is benign or malignant, particularly if it is of an active proliferative papillary type. Complications can include haemorrhage, torsion, infection, rupture, or malignant transformation.

Paraovarian cysts

These arise as remnants of the mesonephric ducts and are lined by a single layer of cubical or columnar epithelium which may be ciliated. The wall is made up of connective tissue, smooth muscle and plastic fibres. These are not strictly true ovarian cysts.

Brenner tumour

This benign fibroepitheliomatous tumour is characterized by the presence of solid and cystic groups of cells showing a wide variation in the proportion of epithelium to connective tissue. They account for 2 per cent of solid ovarian tumours. They resemble a fibroma and have a thick outer fibrous wall which contains microcysts. Microscopic examination reveals clumps or cords of epithelial elements with typical longitudinal grooving. Stroma may be variable in amount and density, and there may be areas of calcification or hyalinization. Very few malignant Brenner tumours have been reported, but they may be associated with Meigs' Syndrome.

EPITHELIAL OVARIAN TUMOURS			
	BENIGN	Borderline (PROLIFERATING)	MALIGNANT
Mucinous	+	+	+
Serous	+	+	+
Endometrioid	rare	+	+
Mesonephroid	rare	rare	+
Brenner	+	rare	rare

Fig. 5.40 Common epithelial ovarian tumours, showing degree of malignancy.

107

Ovarian carcinoma

This may arise as a malignant transformation of a pre-existing tumour or as secondary malignant tumour.

There are three types:

(i) Adenocarcinoma of a well defined type such as mucinous, serous, endometrioid or mesonephroid.

(ii) Adenocarcinoma of unspecified type.

(iii) Undifferentiated carcinoma, consisting of large sheets of epithelial cells showing malignant features but no characteristic pattern.

The prognosis for ovarian tumours, as with all gynaecological malignancies, improves with increasing differentiation of the cells.

The widespread dissemination of tumour throughout the peritoneal cavity, however, accounts for its poor prognosis (Fig. 5.41). The lymphatic drainage is primarily to the para-aortic nodes and within the pelvis. (Fig. 5.42).

Metastatic ovarian carcinoma

This usually arises from three primary sites: (1) gastric; (2) intestinal; and (3) breast. The tumour may appear as nodules on the surface of the ovary or as a well established solid cystic tumour. Often there are bilateral tumours and, if unilateral, the right is more frequently involved than the left. Microscopically they tend to be typical adenocarcinomas or Krukenberg tumours. The tumour cells are usually arranged as clumps of diffusely scattered cells through the stroma and may resemble signet rings in appearance. Other cells are spheroidal and the stroma is richly cellular with spindle-shaped cells. Krukenberg tumours are usually solid and may occasionally be primary.

Spread of metastatic ovarian tumour from the primary may be by surface implantation of seedlings, or via the lymphatics or blood.

Sex cord stromal tumours

Granuloma cell tumours

These are characterized by oestrogenic activity, cells which resemble the granulosa of the Graafian follicle, and a characteristic cell arrangement. The clinical picture varies according to the age of the patient, due to the oestrogenic activity. Postmenopausal patients may present with unexpected bleeding. The size of the tumour can vary from a very small tumour to a large abdominal mass and, although they are usually solid, they may contain a few cysts. Microscopically there is often a mixed pattern of cells which may be luteinized. These tumours are rarely malignant before the menopause. Approximately 25-30 per cent will be malignant at five year follow-up. The longer the duration of follow-up, the higher the proportion of patients who will die from a granulosa cell tumour. They are associated with cystic hyperplasia of the endometrium and occasionally endometrial carcinoma.

Thecoma

This is a tumour structurally resembling a fibroma, but with oestrogenic activity. It may merge with a granulosa cell tumour.

Fibroma

This is a benign connective tissue tumour of common type that is seen in other organs. It accounts for 1.5-5 per cent of all ovarian tumours and occurs most commonly in the elderly, but can occur at any age. Microscopically it looks similar to fibromas seen elsewhere in the body. Secondary changes include oedema, hyalinization, fatty change, haemorrhage, calcification and infarction. Meig's syndrome may occur in association with a fibromas; this comprises ascites and hydrothorax, which disappear on removal of the tumour.

Androblastoma or Sertoli-Leydig cell tumour

This mimics development of the male gonad. Three types are recognized:

(i) Tubular, where the tubules often resemble the Sertoli cells of the testes; there may be androgenic activity.

(ii) Undifferentiated.

(iii) Intermediate.

Eosinophilic cells are frequently present. These resemble interstitial cells of the testes or Leydig cells, and can account for the masculinizing activity of some of these tumours. Malignancy is difficult to evaluate.

Germ cell tumours

These arise from the ovary and may be found to be composed of embryonic structures.

Embryonic tumours

These are otherwise known as teratomas and consists of two types: (1) cystic (dermoid); and (2) solid, which may be composed of mature or immature structures.

Dermoid cysts

These are the most common tumours of young women, but can occur from the first to eighth decade of life. In 10 per cent of cases they are bilateal. They are usually unilocular, filled with fatty material and hair. Sometimes they can contain teeth and various other tissues as they arise from a multipotent cell. Microscopically the tissues present correspond to the three germinal layers, although ectodermal tissue predominates. Complications include torsion, infection, rupture, obstruction of labour, or malignant change.

Solid teratoma

These tend to occur at an earlier age than dermoids. They are usually solid, containing tissues from all three germinal layers which appear in a completely haphazard fashion.

Other germ cell tumours include choriocarcinomas of the ovary or dysgerminomas, but these are relatively rare.

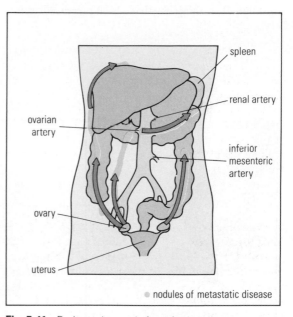

Fig. 5.41 Peritoneal spread of ovarian cancer.

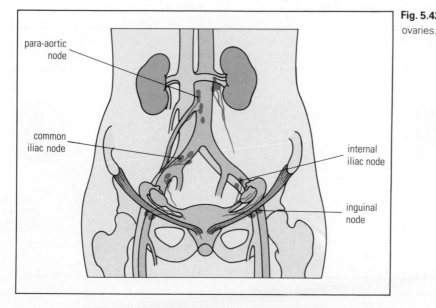

Fig. 5.42 Lymphatic drainage of the ovaries.

Clinical features

Ovarian tumours are often found accidentially, either on abdominal palpation, bimanual palpation, or when using an ultrasound scan to identify another problem. Very large abdominal masses can occur. Sometimes urinary symptoms may result from a large mass pressing on the bladder. In the case of torsion or haemorrhage of the ovarian tumour, the patient will present with pain and sometimes peritonism. Abdominal swelling may have been present for some time, but may be ignored by the patient. There can be a change in menstrual function if oestrogenic or androgen-secreting tumours occur, but in general there is no alteration in the menstrual pattern. In the case of malignant tumours the patient may also have lost weight or become unwell. The differential diagnosis of ovarian lesions is shown in Figs. 5.43 and 5.44.

The clinical staging of malignant ovarian tumours is shown in Fig. 5.45.

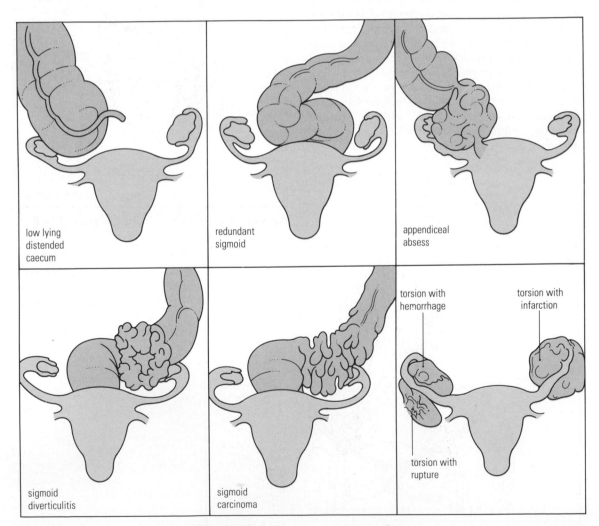

low lying
distended
caecum

redundant
sigmoid

appendiceal
absess

sigmoid
diverticulitis

sigmoid
carcinoma

torsion with
hemorrhage

torsion with
infarction

torsion with
rupture

Fig. 5.43 Differential diagnosis of ovarian lesions.

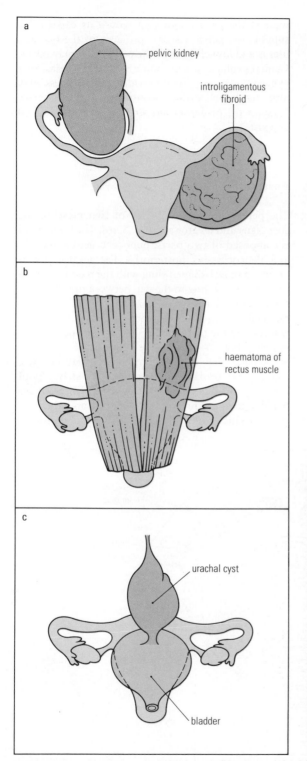

Management

If a patient presents with a ruptured or twisted ovarian cyst, surgery should be performed to untwist the ovary or remove it as appropriate. In the case of malignant tumour, the majority of which are Stage III when diagnosed, surgical management is best with a de-bulking operation, i.e. removing the uterus, both ovaries and tubes, the omentum, and all visible tumour. Peritoneal washings should also be sampled for malignant cells. Even if complete removal of the tumour is not possible, a major reduction in tumour bulk makes chemotherapy and or radiotherapy much more effective. Chemotherapy may be either single or multiagent; one agent should, for preference, be cis-platinum or one of its anologues. Therapy is usually at four-weekly intervals for six courses. If there has been a good response and no residual disease clinically or on CT scan, a second-look operation searching for any evidence of residual disease may be justified. Intraperitoneal chemotherapy may be effective if there is residual tumour which can be surgically removed.

STAGING OF MALIGNANT OVARIAN TUMOURS	
Stage I:	Growth is limited to the ovary or ovaries IA. Only one ovary is involved, with no ascites present IB. Both ovaries are involved, but there is no ascites IC. One or both ovaries are involved and ascites present
Stage II:	Tumour involves one or both ovaries, and pelvic extension is present IIA. Involvement of uterus and Fallopian tubes IIB. Extension to other pelvic tissues
Stage III:	Presence of intraperitoneal metastases
Stage IV:	Distant metastases

Fig. 5.44 Differential diagnosis of ovarian lesions.

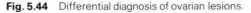

Fig. 5.45 Staging of malignant ovarian tumours.

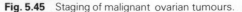

111

Prognosis

In Stage I (which is uncommon) where the growth is limited to either one or both ovaries, the outlook is good with at least an 85 per cent five-year survival rate. Unfortunately, in Stage II disease, where there is evidence of pelvic extension, the five-year survival rate drops to 40 per cent. Stage III disease, which includes the majority of cases despite adequate surgery and combination chemotherapy, has only a two to three-year survival of 30 per cent. Stage IV ovarian malignancy with distant metastases has a very poor prognosis and the majority of patients die within one to two years.

GENITAL PROLAPSE

The floor of the pelvis is composed of muscle and fascia, and is designed to contain the pelvic viscera and to allow childbirth and excretion from the bladder and bowel. In animals which walk on four limbs, there is less gravitational pressure on the pelvic floor from the intra-abdominal contents, but in humans, who have an upright stature, the pressure is greater and the pelvic floor has evolved to contain a larger proportion of fascia to provide more strength. Child-bearing and ageing in particular weaken the pelvic floor and reduce its capacity to support the pelvic viscera; prolapse of the bladder, uterus and bowel through the pelvic floor may result. Genital prolapse is a common source of referral to a gynacologist and, since pelvic floor weakness may also result in stress incontinence of urine (see Chapter 6), prolapse and stress incontinence often co-exist.

Anatomy of the pelvic floor

The pelvic floor is composed of two muscles, the coccygeus and levator ani (Fig. 5.46). The levator ani is composed of two parts, pubococcygeus anteriorly and ileococcygeus posteriorly. The levator ani is arranged in a U-shaped sling with the rectum, vagina and urethra passing in the gap between the muscle in the midline. The anatomical relations are normally retained by fascial attachment between the pelvic vescera and the fascia which envelops the pelvic floor muscle (Fig. 5.47). If the muscle or fascia is weakened, the normal antomical relations will change and prolapse may result. The pelvic floor normally ensures a marked angulation between the bladder and urethra and the rectum and the anal canal. This angulation is important for the

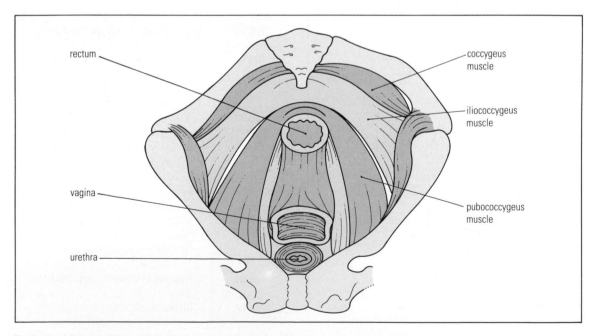

Fig. 5.46 Muscles of the pelvic floor.

maintenance of continence of the bladder and bowel respectively (Fig. 5.48), and so loss of this angulation may lead to loss of urinary or faecal continence.

Uterine supports

In addition to the pelvic floor support, the uterus (and to some degree the vagina) is supported by the round, uterosacral and cardinal ligaments (Fig. 5.49). Weakness of these ligaments will result in prolapse of the uterus and is usually accompanied by pelvic floor weakness, so that uterine prolapse is usually accompanied by prolapse of the bladder (cystocele) and bowel (rectocele or enterocele).

Prolapse of the uterus may be graded according to the level of descent of the cervix in the vagina. In first degree uterine prolapse, the cervix descends to the introitus; in second degree it descends through the introitus, and in third degree prolapse, the whole uterus descends through the introitus (Fig. 5.50). Staging of uterine prolapse is of most value in gauging suitability for surgical removal of the uterus by the vaginal route (vaginal hysterectomy). In general, the greater the degree of uterine descent the easier the operation. Cystocele and rectocele can also be graded but they usually are described as small, medium or large.

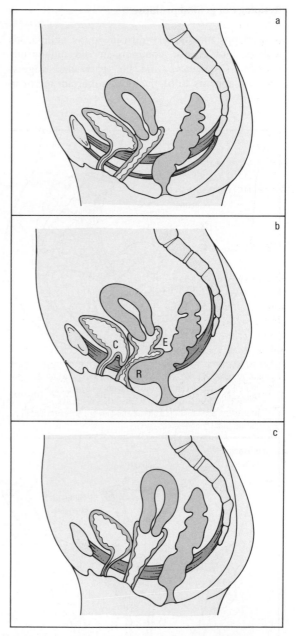

Fig. 5.48 Genital prolapse (top): Normal position; (middle): weak pelvic floor in which the base of the bladder descends below the pelvic floor leading to cystocele (C), the cervix descends, and the pouch of Douglas descends leading to enterocele (E), and the rectum descends, leading to rectocele (R); (bottom): when pelvic floor angulation between the bladder and urethra is weakened, the support of the uterus and vagina and rectum and anal canal are lost.

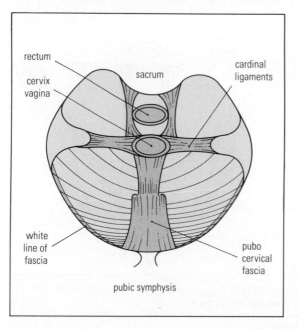

Fig. 5.47 Pelvic fascial supports.

113

Aetiology of genital prolapse

Genital prolapse is very rare in young nulliparous women and is not common in old nulliparous women. Pregnancy, and in particular vaginal delivery, appears to be the most important factor in the aetiology of prolapse. It is not surprising that the pelvic tissues are injured by the passage of a baby through the pelvis; indeed, it is perhaps surprising that all women do not develop prolapse after child-birth. It is not entirely clear why some women

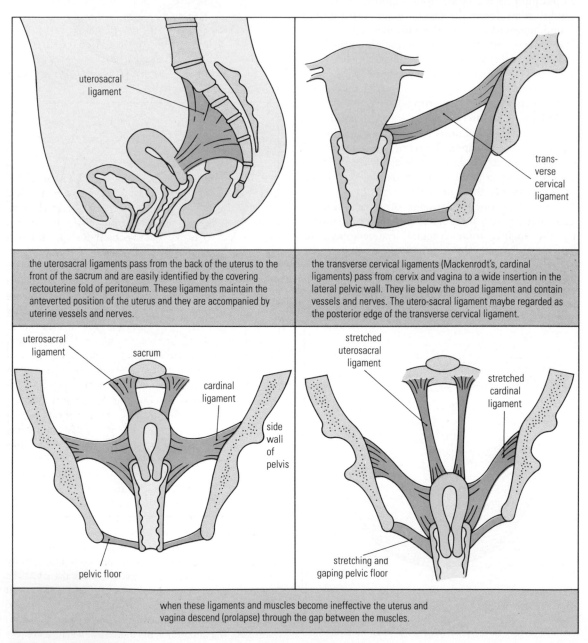

the uterosacral ligaments pass from the back of the uterus to the front of the sacrum and are easily identified by the covering rectouterine fold of peritoneum. These ligaments maintain the anteverted position of the uterus and they are accompanied by uterine vessels and nerves.

the transverse cervical ligaments (Mackenrodt's, cardinal ligaments) pass from cervix and vagina to a wide insertion in the lateral pelvic wall. They lie below the broad ligament and contain vessels and nerves. The utero-sacral ligament maybe regarded as the posterior edge of the transverse cervical ligament.

when these ligaments and muscles become ineffective the uterus and vagina descend (prolapse) through the gap between the muscles.

Fig. 5.49 Ligaments of the uterus.

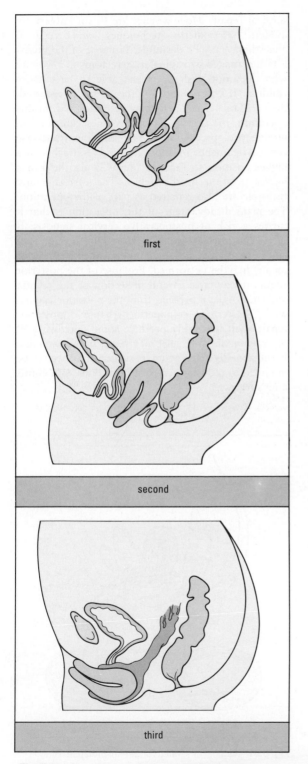

first

second

third

Fig. 5.50 The degrees of uterovaginal prolapse.

are more susceptible than others to prolapse following child-birth, but a long second stage of labour and delivery of a large baby predispose to more pelvic floor injury. All tissues weaken with age, and the pelvic floor is no exception. The lower oestrogen level after the menopause may cause an acceleration of pelvic floor weakness and problems related to prolapse are seen most commonly in postmenopausal women. Conditions associated with elevated intra-abdominal pressure may predispose to genital prolapse because of the additional strain on the pelvic floor. Women who are obese or have a history of a chronic cough are therefore more likely to develop prolapse.

Symptoms of genital prolapse

Relatively severe prolapse may be accompanied by few symptoms. Generally, however, women first become aware of 'something down below'. This tends to become more obvious after prolonged standing, because of gravitational forces, and will therefore be more noticeable later in the day; it may not be a problem in the morning after a night in bed. There may also be low backache, often described as a dragging sensation when the vaginal symptoms are prevalent. Prolapse of the bladder or cystocele may result in urinary symptoms. If the bladder base prolapses and the urethra remains well supported, there may be hesitancy of micturition, frequency and incomplete emptying or even retention. Congestion of the bladder base in a cystocele may increase the sensitivity of the bladder wall, producing frequency, and urgency of micturition. If the cystocele is accompanied by urethral spincter weakness, stress incontinence may occur with abrupt rises in intra-abdominal pressure (see Chapter 6).

Prolapse of the rectum may lead to difficulty in emptying the rectum because a cul-de-sac is produced by the rectocele bulging forward into the vagina. Many women with this problem need to place their fingers in their vagina to aid rectal evacuation. Prolapse of the small bowel through the pouch of Douglas (enterocele: see Fig. 5.48) is rarely severe enough to cause complications, but carries the potentially serious risk of small bowel obstruction through entrapment. Prolapse may cause dyspareunia or apareunia. It is important to discuss this with women, particularly if surgical treatment is contemplated (see below).

Signs of genital prolapse

Examination of a woman who has symptoms of genital prolapse must first involve a careful examination of the abdomen and bimanual examination of the pelvic viscera. An abdominal or pelvic mass may be the underlying cause for a rise in intra-abdominal pressure creating a prolapse. After a bimanual examination in the supine position, the woman is asked to strain down so that the degree of perineal descent or prolapse can be seen. The woman is asked to cough to see if stress incontinence of urine is demonstrable. This may be performed with an empty bladder in the supine position and if stress incontinence is not demonstrable a full bladder and the erect position may be employed. The presence of a cystocele is best demonstrated using a Sims' speculum with the patient in the left lateral position. The speculum is used to hold back the posterior vaginal wall whilst the descent of the anterior wall is visualized at rest and with straining. The descent of the uterus can be visualized in this position. The Sims' speculum may now be rotated through 180° (after withdrawing a little) and the descent of the posterior wall visualized at rest and with straining. It is often difficult to decide whether descent of the posterior vaginal wall posterior to the cervix is enterocele or high rectocele, and the answer may only be revealed at surgery. A finger placed in the rectum will delineate a rectocele.

Treatment of genital prolapse

Treatment depends on the severity of the symptoms, and the age and physical condition of the patient. If the woman wishes to have further children or is unfit for surgery, a conservative approach is required. Conservative therapy involves either pelvic floor physiotherapy, or insertion of a vaginal pessary. Pelvic floor physiotherapy is probably of most value in younger women with mild pelvic floor weakness and prolapse. Some women prefer to avoid surgery, and the prolapse may be supported by a vaginal pessary (Fig. 5.51). When fitted, the woman is not aware of the pessary and must simply return to the doctor every six months so that the vaginal walls may be examined for ulceration. If surgery is requested by a younger woman then it is advisable that further children are delivered by caesarean section since vaginal delivery would damage the

surgical repair. Most women are fit for surgery by modern anaesthetic techniques and regional anaesthesia may be desirable. Prolapse of the uterus is best managed by vaginal hysterectomy in a woman who does not wish or is not able to have more children. If conservation of the uterus is required, then a Manchester repair may be performed. In this operation, the cervix (which becomes elongated in uterine prolapse) is shortened and the transverse cervical ligaments are shortened and re-attached at a higher position so that the uterus is also held in a higher position in the pelvis. The cystocele and rectocele are also repaired as part of the operation. The main disadvantage of this operation is that it carries a risk of postoperative cervical stenosis. If there is sufficient cystocele to require surgery, an anterior colporrhaphy (commonly called an anterior repair) may be performed. Prolapse of the posterior vagina necessitates careful dissection of the rectum and enterocele, if present, from the posterior vaginal wall. Posterior colpoperineorrhaphy (posterior repair) will inevitably produce some narrowing of the vagina which in turn may result in dyspareunia. In the sexually active woman, surgery may need to be modified to reduce the risk of difficulties with coitus after surgery.

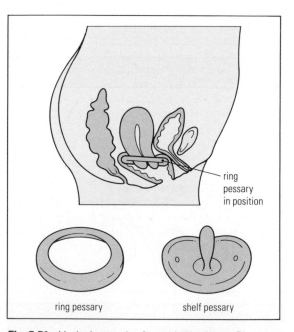

ring pessary in position

ring pessary

shelf pessary

Fig. 5.51 Vaginal pessaries for genital prolapse. Ring pessary (top) and shelf pessary (bottom).

INTRODUCTION

Dysfunction of the lower urinary tract is a common reason for referral to the gynaecologist. The most frequent dysfunction is urinary incontinence which is a debilitating problem both physically and mentally. Ten per cent of women over 15 years of age leak urine twice or more a month and many do not seek medical help, primarily because of embarrassment about their problem.

This chapter will cover the normal function of the lower urinary tract, including the normal mechanism of urinary continence. Disorders of urinary tract function, particularly incontinence, will be discussed, followed by the investigation and management of dysfunction.

NORMAL AND ABNORMAL FUNCTION OF THE LOWER URINARY TRACT

The bladder

Normal control of the bladder
At birth the bladder is emptied by contraction of the detrusor muscle, which is activated by a spinal reflex triggered by stretch receptors in the bladder wall. Between two and four years of age, a supraspinal pathway from the brain matures and enables the child to inhibit the spinal reflex so that micturition can be delayed until a socially convenient time.

Problems with bladder control
The sensitivity of the stretch receptors in the bladder wall may be enhanced by intrinsic factors like inflammatory changes (cystitis) or extrinsic factors like cold weather.This enhanced sensitivity will produce a more frequent desire to pass urine (*frequency*), and may be sufficiently strong to activate the spinal reflex, thereby producing a detrusor muscle contraction which may result in urinary incontinence.

Loss of the capacity to inhibit the spinal reflex may also occur if the supraspinal pathway is injured (e.g. spinal cord injury) and results in the inability to delay micturition. This is known as *urgency*, and may in turn result in *urgency incontinence*. If the spinal reflex pathway is damaged, the contraction stimulus may be lost and the bladder may become atonic. The woman will then be unable to empty her bladder completely which may result in urinary retention with a large distended bladder; several litres may be held in the bladder if both the sensory and motor innervation are damaged. Urine will then leak from the bladder in small quantities when the intravesical pressure becomes greater than the urethral occlusive pressure; this is known as *overflow incontinence*. Overflow incontinence may also occur with peripheral neuropathy in diabetes mellitus and multiple sclerosis, and with drugs with anti-cholinergic side-effects such as Imipramine (an anti-depressant).

Difficulty in bladder emptying may result from either a failure of the bladder to contract, or resistance to emptying in the urethra. In women (unlike men, who often develop prostatic hypertrophy), voiding difficulty is uncommon and if the bladder function is normal, urethral narrowing due to atrophy (see below) or kinking by prolapse are the most common causes. Incomplete bladder emptying will also predispose to urinary infection because of urinary stagnation in the bladder.

The control of the bladder is illustrated schematically in Fig. 6.1.

The urethra

At rest
The urethral lumen is obliterated at rest. The walls of the urethra are held together by the tone generated by the elasticity of the connective tissue, and the smooth and striated muscle sphincters.

During micturition
The smooth muscle of the urethra is in continuity with the muscle of the bladder wall. When the detrusor muscle contracts, the resulting traction on the proximal urethra causes opening of the lumen. This is accompanied by relaxation of the striated muscle

117

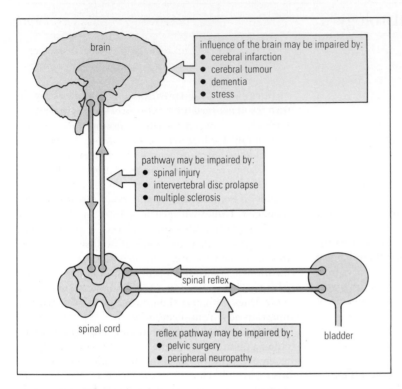

Fig. 6.1 Neural control of the bladder.

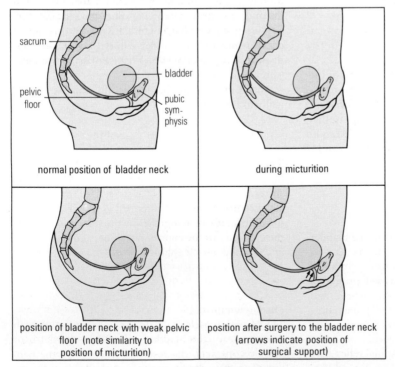

Fig. 6.2 Relaxation of pelvic floor with opening of proximal urethra to allow micturition.

urethral sphincter. Micturition also requires relaxation of the pelvic floor so that the angle between the bladder and urethra is changed to encourage opening of the proximal urethra (Fig. 6.2). Strong contraction of the pelvic floor during micturition will interrupt the flow of urine by changing the urethrovesical angle and possibly by some compression of the urethra.

Under stress

The intra-abdominal pressure rises abruptly when under stress (e.g. coughing, laughing, sneezing). This in turn produces a sharp rise in intravesical pressure. To maintain continence, the urethral occlusive forces must be high enough to overcome the raised intravesical pressure, otherwise urine will leak through the urethra.

The most important parts contributing to urethral occlusion under stress are the striated urethral sphincter and the pelvic floor. The striated urethral sphincter directly occludes the urethral lumen on contraction whilst the pelvic floor maintains the optimum angulation between the bladder and urethra. The effect of weakness of these muscles is illustrated in Fig. 6.2.

Weakness of the striated urethral sphincter and pelvic floor muscles therefore reduces the ability to generate sufficient urethral occlusive forces to overcome raised intravesical pressure during stress; stress incontinence of urine results. Weakness of the striated muscle of the urethral sphincter and the pelvic floor appears to occur with denervation injury during child-birth, and with ageing. This explains why stress incontinence is predominantly found in women who have had children. In some women, the muscle denervation and subsequent weakness is so severe that

prolapse of the rectum (rectocele), bladder (cystocele) and uterus occurs. This explains why stress incontinence of urine and uterovaginal prolapse often co-exist, pelvic floor weakness being the common aetiological factor.

Women who generate a high intra-abdominal pressure (and intravesical pressure) are also more likely to develop stress incontinence of urine. Obese women and women who have a chronic cough are susceptible, and an intra-abdominal mass, e.g. pregnancy or a pelvic tumour, will also contribute to a higher pressure.

The various causes of urinary incontinence are summarized in Fig. 6.3.

Local factors affecting urethral control

The urethra, like the bladder, is prone to inflammatory change. Infection in the urethra (urethritis) will induce a frequent desire to pass urine, pain with passing urine (dysuria), and may also induce urgency of micturition. After the menopause, atrophy of the vaginal epithelium occurs which may result in atrophic vaginitis. Similar changes may occur in the urethra, producing the symptoms of frequency and dysuria, and eventually causing narrowing of the urethra with subsequent voiding difficulty. In most cases topical oestrogens will reverse the changes, but in more advanced cases dilatation of the urethra may be necesssary to overcome the stenosis.

Fistulae as a cause of urinary incontinence

Urinary incontinence may also occur if there is a fistula between the bladder, ureter or urethra and the vagina. The commonest of these fistulae is the vesicovaginal fistula. Urinary fistulae result in the continuous escape of urine into the genital tract from the ureter, bladder, or urethra.

Obstetric urinary fistulae are now uncommon in developed countries because prolonged labour is avoided by early resort to caesarean section. This, unfortunately, is not the case in countries where obstetric facilities are poor. Urinary fistulae are now seen most commonly in this country after pelvic surgery when there has been bladder or uteric injury. Since all these fistulae are relatively uncommon in the UK, they are usually referred to subspecialists in gynaecological urology or to urologists for treatment.

TYPES OF URINARY INCONTINENCE
urgency incontinence
stress incontinence
mixed incontinence (urgency and stress incontinence together)
overflow incontinence
fistula incontinence

Fig. 6.3 Types of urinary incontinence.

The symptoms of the different types of incontinence are summarized in Fig. 6.4.

Psychological factors in urinary incontinence

Function of the lower urinary tract, in common with function of the lower gastrointestinal tract, has subtle links with the psyche. It is well documented that an anxious, introspective individual may express his or her psychological unhappiness with dysfunction of the bladder or bowel, although in many cases it is difficult to determine whether or not the psychological disorder may in fact be secondary to the bladder dysfunction; urinary incontinence is undoubtedly a psychologically debilitating condition.

INVESTIGATION OF LOWER URINARY TRACT DYSFUNCTION

Clinical history and physical examination

In common with investigation of all clinical disorders, a careful history and examination is an essential part of the investigation of the patient with lower urinary tract dysfunction.

Examination must include neurological examination (to exclude peripheral neuropathy or multiple sclerosis) as well as careful pelvic examination. The presence of genitourinary prolapse is relevant, and the patient should be asked to cough in the supine and erect positions to try to demonstrate stress incontinence. Urinalysis to screen for urinary infection and glycosuria is imperative.

History and examination may not reveal the cause of the dysfunction, particularly incontinence, and investigation of the lower urinary tract by urodynamic studies may be required.

Urodynamic studies

Urodynamic studies are designed to assess the function of the lower urinary tract and include those shown in Fig. 6.5.

Micturition chart

The patient keeps a record of each time she passes urine, including the amount passed, and whether incontinence has occured. This provides useful information about bladder capacity and the severity of the incontinence. Ideally, a record of fluid intake should also be recorded.

Measurement of residual volume

After normal micturition, a urethral catheter is passed to establish whether the bladder has been completely emptied. No more than 50ml should remain in the bladder after micturition.

Cystometry

During normal filling of the bladder, there is no pressure rise within the bladder because of the compliance of the bladder walls. The pressure within the bladder during filling can be measured by a pressure transducer in the bladder inserted through the urethra. If a pressure rise of more than $15 cmH_2O$ is

SYMPTOMS OF URINARY INCONTINENCE				
	Urgency incontinence	Stress incontinence	Overflow incontinence	Fistula
Symptoms	frequency urgency	urinary loss with raised intra-abdominal pressure	hesitancy poor stream frequency incomplete emptying	insensible loss
Volume	may be large	small volumes	small volumes	dribble

Fig. 6.4 Symptoms of urinary incontinence.

recorded during filling (which is usually performed with the patient in the supine position, Fig. 6.6), a diagnosis of *detrusor instability* is made. This represents abnormal bladder function and is usually associated with urgency and urgency incontinence.

Cystometry may simply involve measurement of the intravesical pressure during filling. More accurate measurement of the detrusor-generated intravesical pressure is made by measuring the intra-abdominal pressure with a rectal pressure transducer as well. Subtraction of the rectal pressure from the intravesical pressure gives the intrinsic bladder pressure. Further sophistication of the investigation can be introduced by using radio-opaque dye to fill the bladder, and by

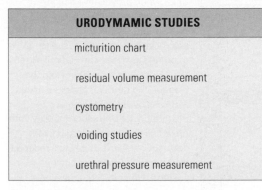

URODYMAMIC STUDIES
micturition chart
residual volume measurement
cystometry
voiding studies
urethral pressure measurement

Fig. 6.5 Urodynamic studies.

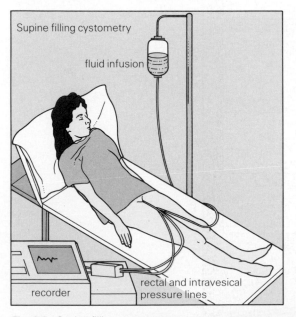

Fig. 6.6 Supine filling cystometry.

screening the bladder radiographically during filling (cystourethrography). If the investigation is recorded on videotape, it can be scrutinized at a later date: this is videocystourethrography (VCU).

Examples of cystometric studies are shown in Fig. 6.7.

Voiding studies

The intra-vesical pressure during voiding, and the voiding urinary flow rate, may be measured. The cause of voiding may be visualized radiographically or surmised from the intravesical pressure and flow rate. A flow rate of at least 20ml per second can normally be achieved.

Urethral closure pressure measurement

Urethral occlusive forces may be measured at rest and during coughing to establish whether they are normal or weak. The advantage of radiographic studies is that leakage of dye into the proximal urethra with straining or coughing can be visualized. Urethral occlusive forces are generally reduced in women who experience stress incontinence of urine.

General points about urodynamic studies

While urodynamic studies are designed to demonstrate dysfunction, they must be interpreted with some caution because of the circumstances in which they are performed. It is not, for example, surprising that many women find it difficult to void in a strange environment with urethral catheters in place and onlookers awaiting urinary flow.

TREATMENT OF URINARY TRACT DYSFUNCTION

Treatment of stress incontinence

The aim of treatment in stress incontinence is to increase the urethral occlusive forces so that they are able to overcome rises in intravesical pressure. For the obese woman it may be sufficient to lose weight, thereby reducing the intravesical pressure generated. Generally, however, treatment is directed towards improving the occlusive forces of the pelvic floor and

121

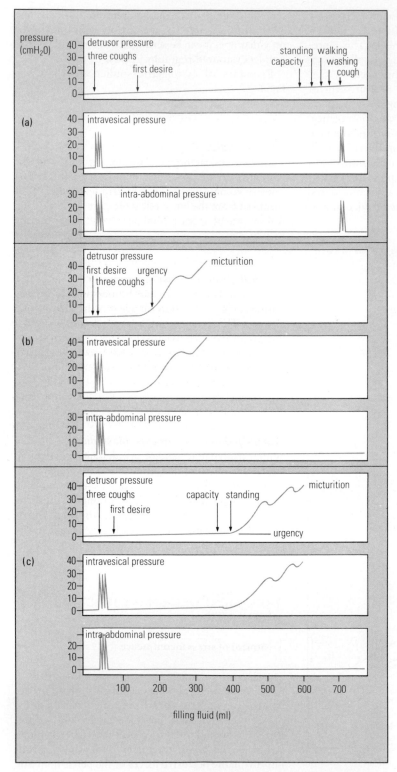

Fig. 6.7 Cystometry studies
(a) Normal cystometry. The diagram illustrates a recording of a three-channel filling cystometry. Fluid is infused at 50ml per minute. Three coughs are recorded by the rectal transducer (intra-abdominal pressure) and the intravesical pressure transducer, but there is no increase in the detrusor pressure. The 'first desire' to micturate is noted here after infusion of 175ml, which is normal. There is no significant rise in detrusor pressure on filling to capacity (5cmH$_2$O). Detrusor contraction are not seen when provocative actions (e.g. standing, hand washing) are performed. (b) Detrusor instability. In this recording, the first desire to micturate is noted early (30ml). After infusion of less than 200ml into the bladder, the detrusor pressure rises and is followed by involuntary micturition. (c) Detrusor instability with provocation. In this recording, the detrusor muscle is stable to a reduced capacity of 375ml in the supine position. On standing, however, detrusor is noted with involuntary micturition.

striated urethral sphincter. Treatment may be conservative or surgical, although most clinicians advocate the use of conservative methods first.

Conservative treatment of stress incontinence

Conservative treatment involves improving pelvic floor and urethral sphincter muscle tone by pelvic exercises.

Active

The pelvic floor is a unique striated muscle in that it is constantly active. Exercising the pelvic floor by voluntary contraction can increase the muscle strength and resting activity or tone. It is particularly important in the postnatal period but is probably advisable antenatally, and as a useful general exercise. Women are advised to try to interrupt their urinary stream by pelvic floor contraction. This ability is commonly lost after child-birth, but may be regained with practice.

Passive

Many women are not able to contract their pelvic floor voluntarily. Direct (Faradism) or indirect (interferential therapy) electrical stimulation of the pelvic floor muscle may help to build muscle strength. It is probable that electrical stimulation is a useful aid in teaching a woman how to contract her pelvic floor rather than as a muscle strength builder.

Surgical treatment of stress incontinence

The surgical treatment of stress incontinence aims to return the proximal urethra to its original position in relation to the bladder and pelvic floor so that rises in intra-abdominal pressure produce a closing rather than an opening force (see Fig. 6.2).

Many operations have been described but no operation is always successful. Surgery may be approached vaginally, abdominally or both. The vaginal approach, referred to variously as an anterior repair or urethral buttress, has the advantage of low morbidity (Fig. 6.8). It has the disadvantage that the surgery effectively takes the 'slack' out of the muscle and fascia around the bladder neck, it relies on the integrity of this tissue for its future strength. Since this tissue is known to weaken with age the vaginal operation probably has a higher recurrence rate than the abdominal approach.

The most commonly adopted abdominal approach to surgery is colposuspension. Dissection behind the pubis through a low transverse abdominal incision gains access to the bladder neck and surrounding fascia from above (Fig. 6.9). The fascia lateral to the

Fig. 6.8 Urethral buttress/anterior repair.

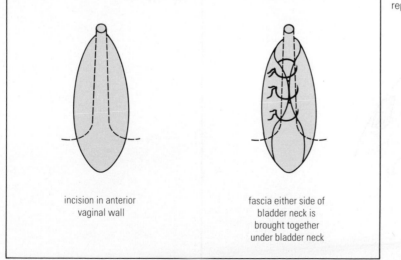

incision in anterior
vaginal wall

fascia either side of
bladder neck is
brought together
under bladder neck

bladder neck is hitched up on each side by sutures which approximate the fascia to the tough, fixed ileo-pectineal ligament on the superior pubic ramus. This operation permits more elevation of the bladder neck than can be gained through a vaginal approach. It is therefore more likely to be effective and gives fascial support to a fixed point which should provide long-lasting strength. This operation does have greater morbidity than the vaginal approach, not only because it necessitates an abdominal incision, which is more painful that vaginal incision, but also because surgery in the cavity of Retzius may be associated with

disturbance of bladder function postoperatively. This may be difficult to treat satisfactorily. A combination of vaginal and abdominal surgery may be used to support the bladder neck with a sling mechanism attached to the rectus sheath of the anterior abdominal wall (Fig 6.10). Strips of rectus sheath fascia are often used for the sling, or denatured pigskin, ox fascia, or synthetic material can be used. Inevitably these operations involving more extensive surgery may produce greater morbidity, but they undoubtedly have a place in carefully selected cases. It is important to advise a patient who is considering surgical treat-

Fig. 6.9 Colposuspension.

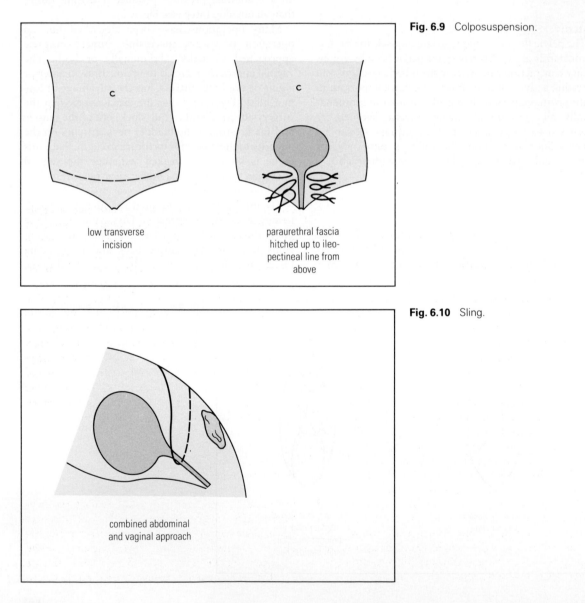

low transverse
incision

paraurethral fascia
hitched up to ileo-
pectineal line from
above

Fig. 6.10 Sling.

combined abdominal
and vaginal approach

ment for stress incontinence that the operation may not cure her condition. Failure to warn her of this before surgery will lead to resentment of failure should it occur and possible medicolegal action.

Postoperative care

Voiding difficulty may be experienced after surgery for stress incontinence. This usually settles within a few days with bladder catheterization. Occasionally the surgery may have to be re-fashioned in order to allow complete micturition.

Since fibrosis is probably not complete until three months after surgery it is imperative that, following surgery for stress incontinence, the minimum strain should be placed on the healing tissues. Any movements which result in an excessive rise in intra-abdominal pressure, e.g. lifting, should be avoided. Since further weakening of the fascia and muscle of the pelvic floor will occur with ageing it is important that, in the long term, women with known weakness of the pelvic floor should avoid activities which are likely to strain the pelvic floor; care with weight gain is also advisable.

Treatment of urgency incontinence

Urgency incontinence produced by detrusor instability is commonly of unknown aetiology. However, if the cause is intervertebral disc prolapse then spinal surgery is required before irreversible damage to bladder innervation occurs.

The main method of treatment of detrusor instability is 'bladder re-training', the object being to re-learn the capacity to inhibit the spinal emptying reflex. This is generally more successful in hospital where it is easier for the woman to concentrate on bladder control without interruptions from routine commitments. Considerable support from nursing and medical staff is also important. Success rates are high initially but regression is common on returning home.

Anti-cholinergic and muscle-relaxant drugs (e.g. Propantheline) may help with bladder re-training. They are often required in doses which are associated with unpleasant side-effect, such as dry mouth, constipation and headaches, which many women find intolerable. No single agent has proved superior and the prescription is generally according to the physician's personal preference.

Stretching the bladder (cystodistension) under general or epidural analgesia is advocated by some clinicians, but there is little evidence to suggest that this procedure provides any long-term benefit.

Treatment of mixed urinary incontinence

When a woman has both detrusor instability and pelvic floor and urethral sphincter weakness, a treatment dilemma emerges. Many physicians prefer to treat the detrusor instability before the stress incontinence since the results from surgery are ofter disappointing when detrusor instability is present. However, bladder re-training is often more difficult if urinary leakage occurs with stress, since urine entering the proximal urethra with a sudden movement will often trigger a contraction from an unstable detrusor muscle. Each case must be treated individually and experience is required to manage such cases.

Treatment of overflow incontinence

Overflow incontinence is uncommon but is easily missed since the symptoms can mimic incontinence produced by other causes. If the cause is outflow obstruction, then this must be relieved, e.g. repair of prolapse. If the cause is bladder atony, or if no treatable cause is found, then management is either with a cholinergic agent such as Distigmine Bromide (which can stimulate contraction of an atonic bladder) or by self-catheterization. The latter is a procedure to which most women initially react unfavourably but they are usually able to manage clean self-catheterization after a few days of sympathetic tuition. The cause of bladder atony must be considered before treatment since, for example, intervertebral disc prolapse may be responsible.

Incontinence aids

Incontinence aids are an important adjunct to care in women with urinary incontinence. They are not only of use in women who have incurable incontinence but also in women undergoing treatment or awaiting treatment. It is imperative in choosing an incontinence aid that the women herself finds the aid acceptable so that she has the confidence to use it and enjoy as normal a life as possible.

The investigation and management of a woman with urinary incontinence is summarized in Fig. 6.11.

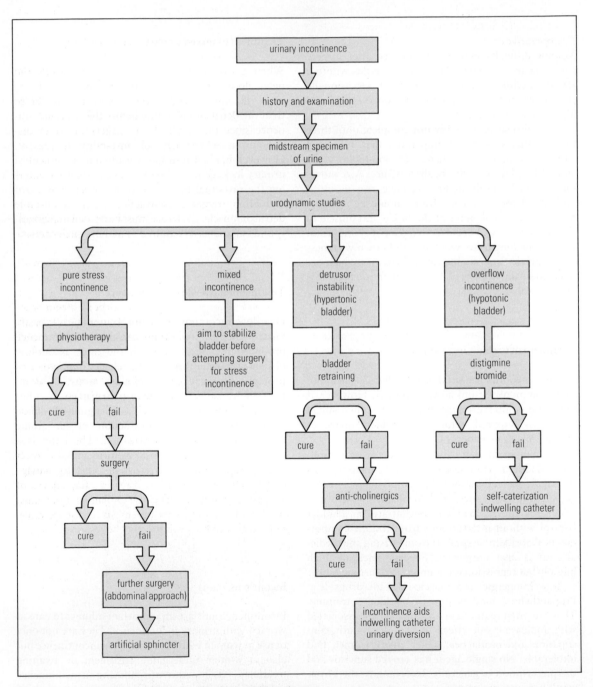

Fig. 6.11 Investigation and management of urinary incontinence.

Gynaecological Imaging

Many methods of imaging are used to demonstrate the reproductive system and the pathology associated with it. Some are relatively simple and others more complex, as enumerated below.

PLAIN X-RAY FILMS

Pelvis

The x-ray film should be taken with an empty bladder, otherwise the bladder might be confused with a pelvic mass.

Demonstrable abnormalities

(i) Soft-tissue pelvic mass with a differential diagnosis of enlarged uterus, ovarian cyst, or tumour.
(ii) Soft tissue calcification may be found in:
(a) Uterine fibroids – typical appearance resembles sponge soaked in barium (Fig. 7.1).
(b) Various benign and malignant ovarian masses, e.g. ovarian dermoid cysts (Fig. 7.2).

(c) The ovaries, which may rarely be completely calcified.
(d) Fallopian tubes – sometimes calcified secondary to tuberculous salpingitis.
(iii) Foreign bodies – intrauterine contraceptive devices (IUCDs), foreign bodies in vagina of children, tampons which have a typical radiolucent, rectangular appearance.

Abdomen

Demonstrable abnormalities

(i) Location of an IUCD which has migrated through the uterine wall into the peritoneal cavity.
(ii) Ascites secondary to ovarian malignancy with peritoneal seeding or ovarian fibroma, and haemoperitoneum secondary to ectopic pregnancy or ruptured corpus luteum may produce a ground-glass, hazy appearance on the radiograph; these are now better detected by ultrasound.
(iii) The distended loops and fluid levels of a paralytic ileus which may occur in association with a ruptured tubo-ovarian abscess.

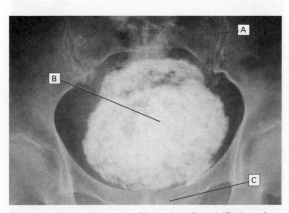

Fig. 7.1 Plain radiograph of large heavily calcified uterine fibroid. (A-sacrum; B-fibroid; C-pubic symphysis).

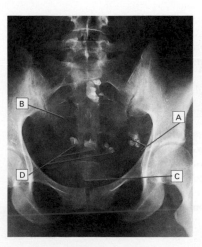

Fig. 7.2 Plain radiograph of ovarian dermoid cyst containing teeth and bone. (A-teeth and bone; B-dermoid; C-compressed bladder; D-teeth).

Chest

Demonstrable pathology
(i) Metastases from pelvic malignancy.
(ii) Tuberculosis, which may be a cause of infertility.
(iii) Pleural effusions associated with Meig's syndrome and disseminated ovarian malignancies.
(iv) Congenital anomalies of the genitourinary tract may also be associated with cardiac abnormalities.

Pituitary Fossa

Chromophobe adenomas of the pituitary gland and craniopharyngiomas may result in increased prolactin levels and therefore may be found in the investigation of amenorrhoea and/or infertility.

Plain photographs of the pituitary fossa (Fig. 7.3) may demonstrate enlargement of the fossa with a double floor, and in the case of a craniopharyngioma, a calcified mass above the fossa.

Computerized axial tomography (CT) scanning will then confirm the diagnosis and show the extent of the tumour (Fig. 7.4).

High-resolution contrast-enhanced CT images with sagittal and coronal reconstruction may be necessary to demonstrate small adenomas which do not enlarge the sella turcica.

Skeleton

Bone metastases occasionally occur, particularly with cervical carcinoma. However, radio-isotope bone scanning is a more sensitive detector of skeletal matastases.

Retarded skeletal maturation and demineralization occurs in Turner's syndrome and in hypopituitarism.

Accelerated skeletal maturation occurs in Albright's syndrome (fibrous dysplasia, café-au-lait spots and precocious puberty). Advanced skeletal maturation also occurs in the adrenogenital syndrome, with enzyme defects in adrenal metabolic pathways, and may occur with secreting gonadal tumours.

CONTRAST EXAMINATIONS

Hysterosalpingography (HSG)

This demonstrates the uterine cavity and Fallopian tubes.

Preparations
The procedure takes place seven days after the end of menstruation, i.e. approximately the 12th day of the menstrual cycle. Effective contraceptive methods should be used in this cycle to avoid irradiating an early fetus.

Method
Up to 10ml of a water-soluble contrast medium is injected into the cervical canal through either a suction type of cannula, a cannula inserted into the cervical os and held in place by volsella forceps, or a Foley catheter held in place by the distended balloon. Normally the uterine cavity and Fallopian tubes are filled and free peritoneal spill occurs from the fimbrial end of the Fallopian tubes. The cannula is removed and a delayed film taken after 20-minute interval.

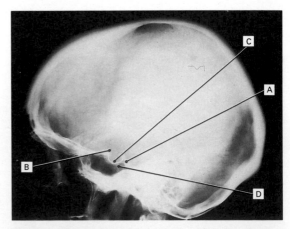

Fig. 7.3 Diagrammatic representation of pituitary fossa on lateral skull radiograph. (A-posterior clinoid processes; B-anterior clinoid processes; C-floor of fossa; D-sphenoid sinus).

Indications

(i) Infertility.

(ii) Recurrent abortion, associated with cervical incompetence or congenital abnormalities of the uterus.

(iii) Confirmation of tubal occlusion following sterilization.

(iv) Demonstration of tubal anatomy prior to attempted reversal of sterilization.

(v) Demonstration of normal genital tract prior to acceptance for AID (artificial insemination by donor).

In the past, HSG was used for the demonstration of a variety of other abnormalities, including fibroids and other uterine and endometrial masses, but it has now been largely superseded by ultrasound and by a fibreoptic techniques such as hysteroscopy.

Contraindications

(i) Pelvic infection: acute salpingitis within the previous six months must be treated before examination; acute vaginitis and cervicitis also need to be treated because of the risk of ascending infection.

(ii) Pregnancy: risk of abortion, teratogenic effect in fetus and, later, increased risk of childhood leukaemia.

(iii) Immediately pre- and post-menstruation: venous intravasation may occur and abscure detailed anatomy.

(iv) Allergy and sensitivity to contrast media: the necessity for the examination above to be reviewed and, if essential, effective steroid cover given.

Complications

(i) Pain (a) Due to instrumentation of cannula, volsella forceps or uterine sound (if necessary). This can be minimized by the use of suction devices.

(b) Pressure of contrast injection: usually associated with tubal spasm or occlusion.

(c) Irritation of pelvic peritoneum by contrast following tubal spill. This frequently causes low-grade pain (like 'period pain') which usually lasts for about for one hour, occasionally up to 24 hours and rarely for several days. Pain is less frequent and less

severe with the latest non-ionic contrast media.

(ii) Pelvic infection: usually this is a exacerbation of exisiting infection and is rarely a new infection.

(iii) Haemorrhage is usually minor and due to trauma to the cervix, and can be reduced by the use of suction devices. Endometrial polyps and carcinoma may bleed.

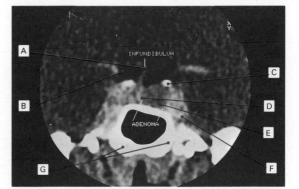

Fig. 7.4 Contrast-enhanced high-resolution CT of pituitary fossa. Corneal section demonstrating microademona. (A-infundibulum; B-basal cistern; C-circle of Willis; D-adenoma; E-pituitary gland; F-cavernous sinus; G-sphenoid bone).

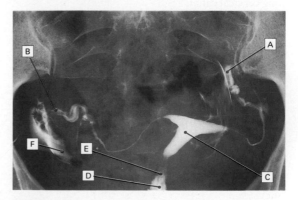

Fig. 7.5 Normal hysterosalpingogram. (A-Fallopian tube; B-fimbrial end of Fallopian tube; C-uterine body; D-cannula; E-cervical canal; F-free spill of contrast from fimbrial end of Fallopian tube into pelvic peritoneum).

129

(iv) Allergic reactions and vasovagal responses are both rare.

(v) Uterine perforation is associated with the use of uterine sounds which are rarely necessary.

(vi) Venous intravasation: when oily contrast media were widely used, this could result in pulmonary or cerebral fat emboli.

(vii) Effect on thyroid function tests: water-soluble contrast can produce elevations of plasma-bound iodine (PBI) for 24-48 hours. Oily contrast (use of which is now rare) produced elevation of PBI for several months.

Normal anatomy (Fig. 7.5)

The uterine body is approximately triangular in shape and 3.5cm in length.

The cervical canal is narrower, and approximately a third of the length of the whole uterus.

The Fallopian tubes are narrow and tortuous, widening to the fimbrial ends from which free spill of contrast into the pelvic peritoneum occurs, producing curvilinear opacities around the bowel loops and in the pouch of Douglas.

Abnormal hysterosalpingogram

Congenital anomalies

In general these are associated with primary infertility or with repeated early spontaneous abortions (see Fig. 2.8).

Infantile uterus: small uterine body and relatively long cervical canal.

Uterine didelphys: reduplication of whole of uterine body, cervix and vagina with single Fallopian tube to each half uterine body.

Uterine bicornis unicollis (bicornuate uterus): reduplication of uterine body with single cervix (Fig. 7.6).

Septate and arcuate uterus: minor degree of reduplication of uterine body.

Unicornuate uterus: single spindly-shaped uterine cavity lying to one side of the midline with a single Fallopian tube. It may or may not have a rudimentary horn (Fig. 7.7).

Uterine masses

These are now usually diagnosed by alternative imaging methods such as ultrasound, hysteroscopy and cytological techniques, etc.

Leiomyomata (Fibroids)

The abnormality depends on the location; often fibroids are multiple and they may then enlarge and distort the uterine cavity, whereas a single submucosal fibroid shows on HSG as a sessile or polypoid filing defect within the uterine lumen.

Carcinoma of the uterine body

This produces a ragged, irregular filling defect.

Pregnancy

Pregnancy produces a smooth, rounded filling defect in the uterus. If the fetus is in a Fallopian tube, the affected side is dilated proximally with abrupt termination at the gestation sac.

HSG is no longer used for the diagnosis of hydatidiform mole or ovarian carcinoma.

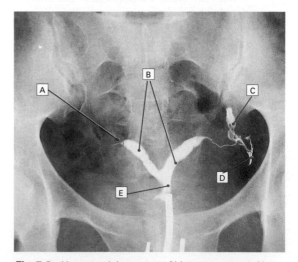

Fig. 7.6 Hysterosalpingogram of bicornate uterus. (A-incompletely filled right Fallopian tube; B-reduplicated uterine body; C-Fallopian tube; D-free spill of contrast; E-single cervical canal).

Salpingitis

Salpingitis may produce:

(i) Tubal occlusion, which results in failure of tubal filling either at the cornua or elsewhere.

(ii) Fimbrial adhesions, which result in failure of contrast to spill freely from the fimbrial end of the tube, and persistence of contrast within the tube on the delayed film.

(iii) Hydrosalpinx, which often results in obstructed and markedly dilated Fallopian tubes (Fig. 7.8).

(iv) Pelvic adhesions, which result in loculation of contrast within the pelvic peritoneum.

(v) Tuberculous salpingitis, which may present simply as obstructed Fallopian tubes, but the tubes may be irregular in calibre, with areas of narrowing and dilatation. Occasionally, calcification is seen in a tuberculous pyosalpinx (Fig. 7.9).

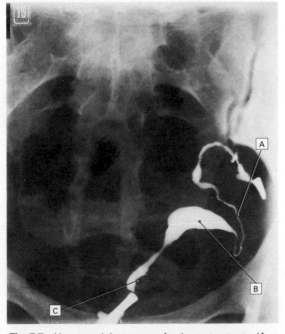

Fig. 7.7 Hysterosalpingogram of unicornate uterus. (A-Fallopian tube; B-single left uterine horn; C-cervical canal).

Confirmation of tubal occlusion following sterilization

The uterine body and proximal portion of both Fallopian tubes are will filled with abrupt tubal obstruction which is often associated with slight dilatation of the terminal portion of the tubes. If present, radio-opaque tubal clips are seen.

Vaginography

Indications

(i) Vaginal fistulae communicating with rectum, bladder or ureter.

(ii) Congenital or acquired vaginal abnormalities.

(iii) Demonstration of ectopic ureter entering the vagina.

Method

Contrast is injected into the vagina through a Foley catheter with the balloon inflated to 30ml, thus obstructing the introitus.

Intravenous urography (IVU)

Indications

(i) Congenital abnormalities of the genital tract: if the anomaly is severe there is a 25 per cent incidence of associated renal anomalies. In many cases this procedure is now replaced by ultrasound.

(ii) Ovarian and uterine masses: demonstration of hydronephrosis, and deviation or compression of the ureters by the mass itself or by associated lymph node metastases.

(iii) Ultrasound will demonstrate hydronephrosis, but not the course of the distal ureter. Computerized tomography (CT) or magnetic resonance imaging (MRI) will demonstrate both and, in addition, will show lymph node metastases.

(iv) Demonstration of ureteric anatomy and renal tract pathology prior to surgery. This is now largely superseded by newer imaging techniques.

(v) Extensive endometriosis may be associated with dilatation of the urinary tract.

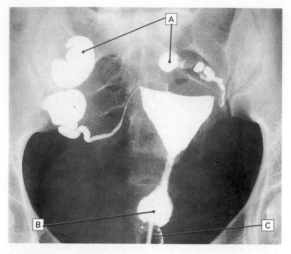

Fig. 7.8 Hydrosalpinx.
(A- obstructed dilated Fallopian tubes; B-cervical canal;
C-cannula).

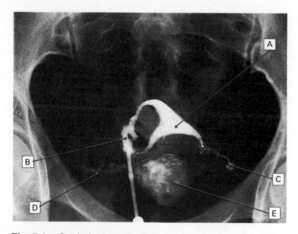

Fig. 7.9 Genital tuberculosis on hysterosalpingogram. (A-anteverted uterine body; B-irregular cervical canal; C-tubal occlusion; D-penetration of contrast between thickened infected mucosa producing an appearance resembling diverticula; E-tuberculous abscess cavity communicating with right Fallopian tube).

(vi) Postoperative ureteric obstruction.
    In the last two conditions, and in other conditions resulting in ureteric obstruction, it is more appropriate to demonstrate the hydronephrosis in the first instance by ultrasound. Isotope renography would then demonstrate renal function. If renal function is adequate, an IVU should then be performed. However if the affected kidney functions poorly, percutaneous antegrade pyelography will demonstrate the level of obstruction precisely, so as to preserve renal function where there is unilateral hydronephrosis or to allow the patient to recover from renal failure where the obstruction is bilateral prior to elective surgery.

Arteriography

Arteriography for the demonstration of pelvic mass lesions been largely superseded by ultrasound, CT, and recently by MRI. However, it still has a role in:
(i)   The demonstration of residual or recurrent tumour where the previous surgery has distorted the normal pelvic anatomy.
(ii) A therapeutic role in selective embolism of tumour.
(iii) A therapeutic role in selective placement of a catheter in the internal iliac artery to facilitate continuous infusion of cytotoxic agents.

Iliac phlebography

The venous drainage of the pelvic organs may be demonstrated by direct injection of contrast into both femoral veins, or interosseous injection into both the greater trochanter and the pubic bones.

Ovarian phlebography

A catheter is introduced into the femoral vein and the ovarian veins are selectively catheterized. The left ovarian vein enters the left renal vein, and the right ovarian vein enters the inferior vena cava (IVC) below the level of the renal veins.

Indications
Demonstration of the extent of known neoplastic disease of the female genital tract and its effect on the venous system including the IVC.

Pelvic phlebography

Pelvic phlebography may demonstrate:
(i)   Complete venous occlusion.
(ii) Narrowing due to extrinsic compression or intramural thrombus.
(iii) Presence of intrapelvic or extrapelvic collateral veins secondary to obstruction, e.g. the presacral plexus or perineal veins.
(iv) Stasis, with reflux of contrast down the ipsilateral leg veins.

Uterine phlebography

Indications
Suspected pelvic varicocele, e.g. in women with chronic pelvic pain and negative investigations.

Contraindications
Pelvic inflammatory disease; menstruation.

Technique
A transvaginal, transuterine approach is used. The cannula is inserted into the myometrium, and hyaluronidase is injected five minutes prior to contrast injection.

If positive, the injected contrast demonstrates dilated, tortuous uterine and ovarian veins.

Lymphography

Indications
Lymphography is indicated to search for spread of secondary tumour to regional lymphatics before surgery or planning of the treatment field, and before radiotherapy in women with pelvic malignancy.

The inguinal, iliac and para-aortic lymph nodes may be demonstrated by injection of the oily contrast medium lipiodol directly into the lymphatics of the dorsum of each foot.

The value of lymphography is limited by the failure to demonstrate hypogastric, paracervical, obturator and presacral lymph nodes reliably; however, these areas are usually included in the radiation field anyway. Lymphography is therefore used to detect spread or recurrence outside the pelvic cavity.

Careful monitoring is necessary during contrast injection because of the danger or oil embolism.

Although CT is widely used for demonstration of both the primary tumour and secondary spread, lymphography is capable of demonstrating infiltrated but non-enlarged nodes, which are undetectable by CT. These nodes have a 'moth-eaten' appearance. In spite of this, in most centres, lymphograpy has been superseded.

Contrast remains in the nodes for a variable time – between six weeks and two years. Therefore while it remains plain films of the abdomen and pelvis may be useful to monitor response to treatment.

Lymphocysts, which occur quite frequently after major pelvic surgery, may be demonstrated when contrast enters the cystic spaces, but are more conveniently demonstrated by ultrasound.

ULTRASOUND

Full knowledge of relevant clinical details is essential to obtain an accurate ultrasonic diagnosis, as various gynaecological pathologies may give a simular ultrasonic appearance, e.g. endometriosis and tubo-inflammatory masses may mimic ectopic pregnancies.

Methods of scanning

Real-time
(i) Transabdominal approach through a full bladder. (The full bladder, by displacing gas-filled loops of intestine which would interfere with the transmission of ultrasound, acts as an acoustic window to visualize the reproductive organs.)
(ii) Transvaginal approach: the bladder is empty and no preparation is necessary. This approach uses higher frequency probes with resultant improved image resolution. However, only structures within 8cm of the transducer are clearly visualized. Increasing use of this method should improve the specificity of gynaecological ultrasound.

Doppler ultrasound

The pulsed Doppler technique using the transvaginal probe enables the operator to make quantitative measurement of blood flow in the ovarian vessels.

Uses of ultrasound

(i)   Demonstration of pelvic masses, their size and origin and their associated secondary effects, such as hydronephrosis, ascites and intra-abdominal metastases.

(ii) Investigation of infertility, e.g. polycystic ovaries.

(iii) Assessment of ovarian follicle development for donor insemination (DI), hormone therapy or *in vitro* fertilization (IVF).

(iv) Demonstration of presence or absence of IUCD within the uterus.

(v)   Ectopic pregnancy.

(vi) Investigation of paediatric or adolescent patients where clinical examination is inappropriate or impossible.

(vii) Ultrasound-guided interventional procedure, e.g. oocyte retrieval for IVF, percutaneous fine-needle aspiration biopsy, drainage of fluid collections, or percutaneous nephrostomy.

Normal anatomy

On transabdominal scanning, the uterus lies posterior to the bladder (which is anechoic) in the midline and has a uniformly fine echopattern (Fig. 7.10). In the mature nulliparous woman, the uterus is up to 7cm in length, and 4cm in anteroposterior and transverse measurements.

The endometrium is seen as a brighter, central-cavity echo which undergoes changes during the menstrual cycle. A characteristic low-density halo is seen around the bright echoes of the endometrium in the preovulatory phase and this can assist in determining the time of ovulation.

The vagina is seen as an echogenic line surrounded by the thin, relatively hypoechoic, muscular wall.

Normal Fallopian tubes and broad ligaments are only rarely seen but 99 per cent of ovaries are demonstrable (Fig. 7.11). They are variable in location, and pulsations in the internal iliac and ovarian arteries assist in locating them. The normal mature ovary measures 3cm (transverse) by 1cm (anteroposterior) by 1cm in height, and normal ovarian volume is 2-6cm^3 (calculated from the formula for a prolate ellipse where volume, $V = 0.52333 \times D_1 \times D_3 \times D_3$, (length, width and breadth). The ovary is usually slightly hypoechoic compared with the uterus, and the developing follicle is seen as an anechoic, cystic structure with a daily increase in size until ovulation. Later the corpus luteum is seen.

Pelvic masses

Real-time ultrasound demonstrates the location, structure (i.e. solid, cystic or mixed) and size of pelvic masses, but often will not demonstrate reliably their pathological nature, although, in general, the more ultrasonically complex the mass the greater the likelihood of malignancy. Doppler ultrasound may in future facilitate a more accurate diagnosis.

Uterine fibroid (Fibromyomata) (Fig. 7.12)

Uterine fibroids may be single and discrete, or multiple, producing a lobulated uterine outline and possibly massive enlargement. They are usually slightly less dense than the uterus and, when calcified, contain highly echogenic foci with distal

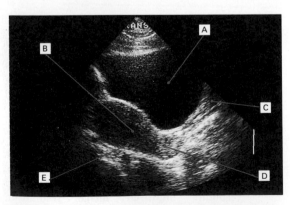

Fig. 7.10 Ultrasound scan of normal mature anteverted uterus – visualization is facilitated by the full bladder which acts as an acoustic window. (A-bladder; B-echo-genic endometrium; C-vagina; D-uterine cervix; E-uterus).

acoustic shadowing. Echo-free areas may result from red degeneration, but cannot be reliably distinguished from sarcomatous change. They may become echo-poor in pregnancy. Pedunculated subserous tumours may be difficult to differentiate from adnexal masses.

Hydatidiform mole (Fig. 7.13)

This characteristically presents as a 'snow-storm' appearance owing to the reflective surfaces of the vesicles of the mole. Coexistence of lutein cysts may indicate progression to choriocarcinoma, but this is not inevitable and no specific criteria for malignancy are available. Diagnosis of blighted ova and missed

abortion by ultrasound, with resultant earlier evacuation, has resulted in a reduced incidence of hydatidiform moles and choriocarcinoma.

Benign ovarian cysts

Benign ovarian cysts, e.g. serous cystadenoma, ultrasonically contain no internal echoes apart from an occasional thin septal wall. They are vary variable in size, and large unilocular cysts may be mistaken for the bladder unless the patient is scanned with a full bladder.

Dermoid cysts (Fig. 7.14)

Dermoid cysts have a mixed internal structure. Features which assist in diagnosis are layering of hair, fat and sebum within the tumour, or inverse layering whereby the solid elements 'float' on the cystic elements. Acoustic shadowing is frequently seen, associated with hair and sebum or with bones and teeth within the cyst. Small echo-dense cysts may be difficult to distinguish from adjacent bowel. The tumour is ill-defined in the two per cent of patients in whom malignancy has occurred, and then there is often demonstrable lymphadenopathy.

Because of the markedly varying density within the tumour, ovarian teratomas are readily diagnosed by CT.

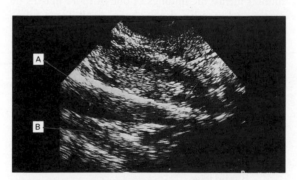

Fig. 7.11 Transvaginal scan of normal right ovary containing three immature follicles (arrowed). (A-iliac vein; B-right iliac artery).

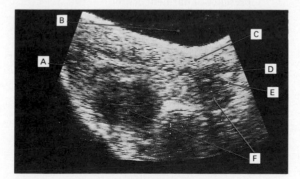

Fig. 7.12 Ultrasound or uterine fibroids. (Two hypoechoic masses involving the posterior uterine wall: longitudinal scan). (A-uterine fundus; B-bladder; C-normal uterine echoes; D-endometrial echoes; E- uterine cervix; F- uterine fibroids).

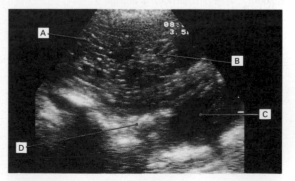

Fig. 7.13 Hydatidiform mole. Enlarged uterus contains numerous echoes and some visible vesicles. Snow-storm appearances. (A-uterus; B-hydatidiform miles; C-theca lutein cyst; D-gas in bowel loops with distal acoustic shadowing).

Maligant ovarian cysts (Fig. 7.15)

Ultrasound will detect even small cystic masses and the majority of malignant ovarian tumours are in part cystic.

When small, however, it is impossible to differentiate benign from malignant ovarian cysts using real-time ultrasound alone. However, Doppler ultrasound has recently been described as being of value in making this distinction, as the neo-vascularization associated with malignant tumour growth results in increased blood flow.

Large tumours, if predominantly cystic, contain thick and irregular septa; if predominantly solid, they usually contain some cystic areas.

Ascites is readily seen with ultrasound and may be massive, although it is not specific for malignancy as it may occur in association with ovarian fibroma in Meig's syndrome. In the presence of ascites, subdiaphragmatic tumour seedlings may be seen.

Hepatic secondaries or hydronephrosis secondary to ureteric obstruction may be seen.

In spite of this, ultrasound is best used as the initial examination to confirm the diagnosis of maligant ovarian cyst, but CT is a more accurate method than ultrasound in staging the tumour.

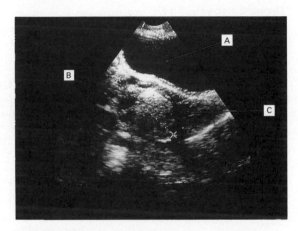

Fig. 7.14 Oblique scan of left ovary demonstrating an ovarian dermoid which is highly echogenic due to sebum hair, etc (incidental finding in asymptomatic patients). (A-bladder; B-ovarian dermoid; C-uterus).

Miscellaneous extrauterine masses

Similar ultrasonic findings of one or more masses of cystic or low-echo density may result from tubo-ovarian abscess (Fig. 7.16), hydrosalpinx (Fig. 7.17), endometriosis or ectopic pregnancy. Therefore, knowledge of relevant clinical details is essential.

Ultrasound findings

Pelvic inflammatory disease

(i)   Free pelvic fluid, resulting in distinct organ boundaries.

(ii) Pyosalpinx and tubo-ovarian abscess: both conditions present as cystic and low-density adnexal masses containing echoes due to the presence of purulent debris

(iii) Hydrosalpinx: anechoic serous fluid.

(iv) Pelvic adhesions with loculated collection of pelvic fluid.

The role of the ultrasound in pelvic inflammatory disease is:

(i)   To gauge the effectiveness of treatment.

(ii) To demonstrate development of complications such as hydrosalpinx or pelvic abscess.

(iii) To help elucidate the cause of infertility.

Endometriosis

Ultrasound is not of value in making the primary diagnosis of endometriosis because the diffuse form with multiple pelvic implants may be difficult to

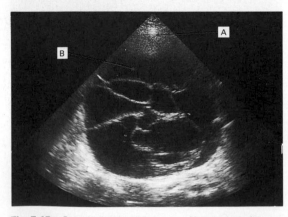

Fig. 7.15 Cystadenoma of the ovary. (A-reverberation artifact; B-ovarian mass).

identify sonographically, and the sonographic features of endometriosis are non-specific. However, it is of some value in assessing response to treatment or recurrence of endometriosis which present as with cystic or low-echo density pelvic masses in which diffuse low-level echoes may be seen universally dispersed with swirling of cyst material during palpation or sudden change of position.

Investigation of infertility

Ultrasound is used:

(i) Demonstration of the presence of a normal uterus and ovaries: although it is possible to demonstrate uterine anomalies, e.g. bicornate uterus on ultrasound, HSG may be more helpful.

(ii) Demonstration of normal follicular development (see next section).

(iii) Demonstration of polycystic ovaries.

(iv) Demonstration of tubal pathology, but again this is more reliably demonstrated by other techniques such as HSG (as previously described).

Ultrasound features of polycystic ovaries (Steinleventhal syndrome) (Fig. 7.18).

(i) Bilateral ovarian enlargement, often rather spherical. Ocasionally only one ovary is enlarged.

(ii) Multiple small cysts, less than 10mm in diameter are often seen around the periphery of the ovary, but are sometimes dispersed throughout.

(iii) Increased echodensity of the ovarian stroma.

Ectopic pregnancy (Fig 7.19)

Typical ultrasound findings are:

(i) Absence of intrauterine pregnancy.

(ii) Sight uterine enlargement and thickened endometrium.

(iii) Adnexal mass, which may be cystic or hypoechoic, and in which there may or may not be a demonstrable gestation sac and fetus.

(iv) Free fluid in the pouch of Douglas.

These findings, plus a positive pregnancy test, are highly specific. However, not all ectopic pregnancies are visualized on transabdominal ultrasound.

The demonstration of intrauterine pregnancy does not exclude the presence of a co-existing ectopic and it should be noted that, with the increasing use of hormonal induction of ovulation, the overall incidence has increased from one in 30000 to one in 7000 pregnancies.

Transvaginal scanning facilitates earlier diagnosis of ectopic pregnancies at a stage where relatively minor surgical intervention such as translaparosopic removal of the gestation sac is possible. Ultrasound-guided transvaginal needle aspiration of early ectopic pregnancies is possible.

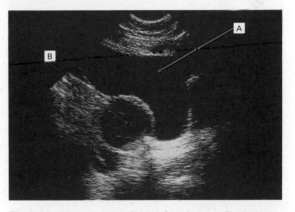

Fig. 7.16 Mass due to tubo-ovarian abscess displacing both uterus and bladder (longitudinal ultrasound scan). (A-bladder; B-ovarian abscess).

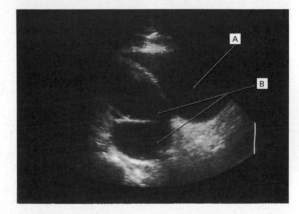

Fig. 7.17 Hydrosalpinx – longitudinal ultrasound scan to right or midline demonstrating the bilocular cystic structure of a dilated tortuous right Fallopian tube. (A-bladder; B-hydrosalpinx).

137

Ultrasound of paediatric and adolescent patients
Indications

(i) Screening for genital anomalies in children with known anorectal or renal anomalies, e.g. there is a 70 per cent incidence of genital anomalies such as bicornate uterus in association with unilateral renal agenesis.

(ii) Demonstration of pelvic organs in infants with anomalous or ambiguous genitalia.

(iii) Primary or secondary amenorrhoea.

(iv) Precocious puberty: search for functioning ovarian tumour.

(v) Possible pelvic mass, e.g. haematometra or haematocolpos.

(vi) Possible pelvic abscess.

(vii) Vaginal discharge: look for foreign bodies in vagina.

(viii) Pelvic pain.

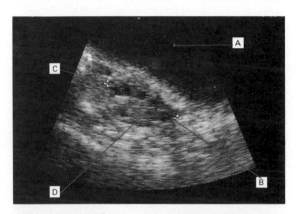

Fig. 7.18 Polycystic ovary. (A-bladder; B-enlarged polycystic ovary (>6cm^3); C-multiple small cysts (often seen around the periphery of the ovary but may be distributed throughout); D-increased stromal echoes resulting in hyperechoic stroma).

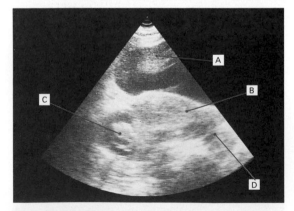

Fig. 7.19 Intra-abdominal ectopic pregnancy at 12 weeks. Placenta seen to be attaching to both uterine fundus and loop of intestine on ultrasound scan; viable fetus. Blood in cul-de-sac. (A-bladder; B-uterus; endometrium; C-foetus; placenta; D-free fluid in cul-de-sac).

Assessment of ovarian follicle development

Ultrasound is useful in evaluation of ovarian function as both follicular measurement and corpus luteum formation can be monitored (Fig. 7.20).

Ovarian scanning is indicated during spontaneous cycles to assist in prediction of ovulation in patient undergoing artificial insemination. Variability of follicular size means that ovulation cannot be precisely timed by follicular measurement alone. However, using vaginal scanning the dissociated oophorus can be seen in an increasing proportion of patients. This indicates that the LH surge has occurred, and so ovulation is probable within the next 24 hours.

The appearance of the endometrium varies throughout the cycle and may also be used to predict the timing of ovulation.

During stimulated cycles the role of sonography is to:

(i) Detect the number of developing follicles.

(ii) Assess the adequacy of follicular response.

(iii) Detect ovulation.

(iv) Assist in timing the administration of HCG.

(v) Detect complications.

As in spontaneous cycles, patients are scanned daily from day nine.

Ultrasound demonstrates those cases with poor follicular development and provides information about defective ovulation where cysts fail to decrease in size after spontaneous LH surge or HCG administration.

Hyperstimulation is characterized by multiple follicles and development of luteal cysts before ovulation, so that treatment may be abandoned because of the chance of multiple pregnancy if artifical insemination is carried out (Fig. 7.21).

Severe hyperstimulation is life-threatening and is characterized by marked ovarian enlargement, up to

10cm in diameter, and by the presence of peritoneal and pleural effusions.

Ovarian ultrasound, together with the assessment of oestradiol levels, may be used to predict patients in danger of developing this condition. If HCG is then withheld, the full expression of the condition is avoided.

Ultrasound imaging of intrauterine contraceptive devices (IUCD)
Indications
(i) 'Lost coil', when the threads are no longer palpable and therefore may be misplaced or lost externally.

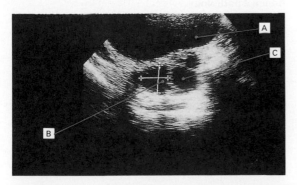

Fig. 7.20 Ultrasound of stimulated ovary demonstrating developing Graffian follicles. (A-bladder; B-Graffian follicles; C-ovary).

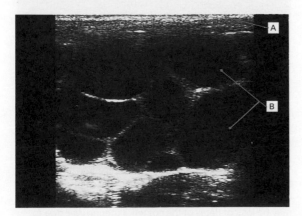

Fig. 7.21 Ultrasound scan (linear array) of hyperstimulated ovary. (A-abdominal wall; B-multiple enlarged Graffian follicles).

(ii) Confirmation of correct placement: this is not routine, but is helpful in patients at risk from misplacement, e.g. obese or postpartum patients.
(iii) Method failure and confirmation of pregnancy.

Ultrasound appearances of IUCD (Fig. 7.22)
The IUCD is highly reflective with distal acoustic shadowing. Differential diagnoses include echogenic premenstrual endometrial echo pattern, retained bone fragments from incomplete abortion, and fibroid calcification.

If properly placed, the IUCD is situated in the fundal area of the cavity and is entirely distal to the internal cervical os.

Complications
The IUCD may perforate the uterus and, if the perforation is complete, the uterus is sonographically empty with radiographic evidence of the IUCD in the pelvis or occasionally the abdomen.

If partial perforation has occurred, a portion of the device is seen embedded in the myometrium

X-RAY COMPUTED TOMOGRAPHY (CT) AND MAGNETIC RESONANCE IMAGING (MRI)

CT is a non-invasive technique which requires some initial preparation of the patient. It displays its clinical image as a body cross-section, generally obtained at 2-3cm intervals moving from the symphysis pubis upwards. The scan is easy to perform and to interpret and has high tissue specificity and image resolution. However, it is expensive and it has a relatively high dose of ionizing radiation which is an important consideration, especially in younger patients.

MRI produces excellent anatomical detail in multiple planes both in normal and pathological conditions and will delineate blood vessels without the use of contrast. It allows a larger field of view than ultrasound, it is not operator-dependent, and it is less affected by bowel gas and body build. Unlike computed tomography (CT) scanning it does not use ionizing radiation or suffer from the image degradation caused by bony structures. However, its use is limited because it is time-consuming and even more expensive than CT, and it cannot be used in patients with certain metal implants such as vascular intracranial clips and pacemakers. At present, its use is confined to selected cases, and it is not a primary imaging method. The planes and images for gynaecological purposes are as follows:

Sagittal plane: demonstrates cephalocaudal tumour extension and best demonstrates vesical and rectal involvement.

Transverse plane: demonstrates lymph node enlargement

Transverse and coronal images are recommended for ovarian pathology and uterine fibroids (leiomyomas).

Uterine pathology

Whilst MRI has a 92 per cent sensitivity for detection of leiomyomas, ultrasound remains the primary imaging method.

Endometrial carcinoma

This cannot be consistently distinguished from blood clot, submucosal degenerative fibroid, or adenomatous hyperplasia, but once endometrial carcinoma has been diagnosed histologically, local staging of the disease is excellent with an overall accuracy of 82 per cent in distinguishing superficial from deep myometrial invasion. It may ultimately replace CT for this purpose. Neither MRI nor CT can distinguish between malignant and hyperplastic lymph nodes.

Cervical carcinoma

MRI is superior to CT as it has superior contrast resolution in demonstrating the cervix, vagina and uterine zonal anatomy, whereas CT cannot consistently separate tumour from the surrounding cervical or parametrial tissue and cannot reliably demonstrate uterine or vaginal involvement. MRI cannot, however, differentiate malignant cervical neoplasia from postbiopsy changes, inflammatory

disease, or, sometimes, enlarged Nabothian follicles or cysts; histology therefore remains essential for the initial diagnosis. It is not indicated for all patient, but is invaluable in assessment of those women with carcinoma of the cervix diagnosed in pregnancy because it does not use ionizing radiation.

Recurrent pelvic tumour

Unlike CR, MRI can be distinguish recurrent tumour from postoperative fibrosis, but has limited value in separating chronic inflammation from recurrent tumour.

Adnexal pathology

The large field of view of MRI and its detailed anatomical delineation facilitates the demonstration of the site of origin of a pelvic mass, but MRI cannot distinguish between benign and malignant tumour. The role of MRI in the demonstration of ovarian malignancies is not fully assessed and CT remains the method of choice for staging ovarian neoplasms.

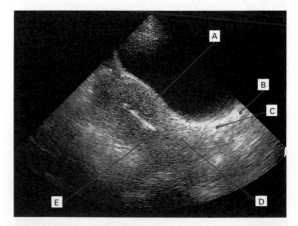

Fig. 7.22 Intrauterine contraceptive device positioned correctly within the uterus on ultrasound scanning. There may be loss of detail of the posterior uterine wall due to acoustic shadowing distal to the IUCD. (A-highly reflective echoes of copper 7 IUCD. B-vagina; C-uterine cervix; D-endometrial echoes; E- uterine body).

INTRODUCTION

Hormone therapy has been used for many years in gynaecological conditions. It is also used in a number of non-gynaecological conditions, e.g. the use of oestrogen in carcinoma of the prostate. The introduction of the combined oral contraceptive pill led to an increased and more widespread use of hormone therapy in premenopausal and postmenopausal women for the treatment of symptoms, as well as prevention of osteoporosis. The interest of the popular media has particularly focused on this last use, and it is likely that hormone therapy will be increasingly used.

The main categories where hormone therapy is used are:
- (i)   Infertility.
- (ii) Contraception.
- (iii) To control menstrual symptoms.
- (iv) Miscellaneous symptoms.

The hormones most commonly used in hormone therapy are oestrogens and progesterones.

PHARMACOLOGY

Oestrogens

Oestrogens used for hormone therapy can be classed into two main groups: natural oestrogens such as oestradiol and oestriol; and synthetic preparations including ethinyl oestradiol, mestranol and stilboestrol. Synthetic oestrogens have not been shown to have any appreciable disadvantages and ethinyl oestradiol is the oestrogen of choice for treating most conditions. All oral preparations are subject to first-pass metabolism in the liver and gut, so subcutaneous or transdermal administration more closely mimics endogenous hormonal activity. Most common available oral preparations use synthetic oestrogens.

Progesterones

Progesterones are also available as natural and synthetic preparations. Dydrogesterone and medroxyprogesterone are found naturally, whereas norethisterone, a commonly used progesterone, is a synthetic testosterone analogue. Progesterone and its analogues are less androgenic than natural testosterone, which can have serious virilizing effects, including a permanent change of voice.

Other preparations

Other preparations work by decreasing androgenic activity. Sebum secretions are decreased by reducing androgen production. Anti-oestrogens include clomiphene, cyclofenil and tamoxifen, which are used in treating infertility and oestrogen-sensitive breast cancer. They induce gonadotrophin releasing hormone (GnRH), which occupies oestrogen receptors in the hypothalamus, thereby interfering with feedback mechanisms. Gonadotrophins such as follicle stimulating hormone (FSH) and human chronic gonadotrophin (HCG) are also used in the treatment of infertility, as is buserelin, a GnRH analogue. This causes an initial stimulation of luteinizing hormone (LH) release and subsequent inhibition, the inhibition resulting from increased testosterone production (in both women and men). Bromocriptine is a stimulant of dopamine receptors in the brain and inhibits the release of prolactin by the pituitary. It is used in infertility, and to suppress lactation. Anti-androgens such as cyproterone acetate may be used to treat acne or hirsutism in women. Danazol is used in the management of endometriosis and acts by inhibiting pituitary gonadotrophin secretion.

INFERTILITY

Infertility caused by defective or absent ovulation may occur as a result of hypothalamic pituitary dysfunction or hyperprolactinaemia, and it is in these cases that hormone therapy is used to induce ovulation. A careful history must be taken, including drug therapy and the length or irregularity of the menstrual cycle, followed by a careful examination. The menstrual cycle pattern may suggest the diagnosis, e.g. oligomenorrhoea or oligomenorrhagia in polycystic ovarian syndrome. Prolactin levels and FSH:LH ratios should be measured in all patients, as well as luteal serum progesterone and testosterone, where appropriate. Very high levels of gonado-trophins are found in patients with premature menopause or the resistant ovarian syndrome. Testosterone may be raised in those with polycystic ovaries. A summary of the hormonal causes, diagnoses and possible treatments of infertility in the anovulatory patient is given in Fig. 8.1.

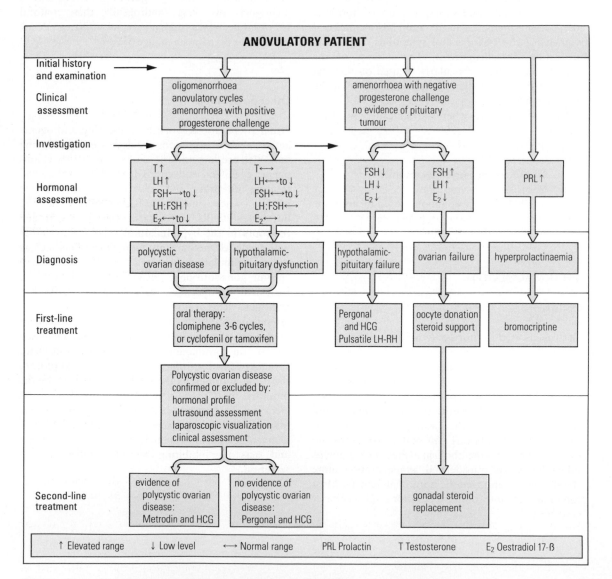

Fig. 8.1 Diagnosis and induction of ovulation in the anovulatory patient.

Hyperprolactinaemia

If prolactin is found to be significantly raised on two occasions, then treatment with bromocriptine can be commenced, once a pituitary tumour has been excluded by visual field testing and pituitary fossa X-ray. Side-effects of bromocriptine include nausea, vomiting and occasionally postural hypertension. Most women become tolerant of these, but very high doses can cause peptic ulceration. Therapy is stopped as soon as pregnancy is confirmed, although there is no evidence that bromocriptine causes fetal abnormalities. After pregnancy and breast feeding, prolactin levels should be checked at regular intervals as treatment may need to be recommended.

Anovulation with normal prolactin levels

Anovulation where prolactin levels are normal may be due to a variety of causes:
  (i) Premature menopause, where treatment is rarely successful.
  (ii) Polycystic ovarian disease, where success with treatment is usually good.
  (iii) Post–pill amenorrhoea which usually resolves spontaneously with time.
  (iv) Hypothalamic amenorrhoea where the results are variable.

If the patient is amenorrhoeic, a progesterone challenge test with medroxyprogesterone acetate 5mg twice daily for four days is given to see if bleeding occurs. This indicates whether the endometrium can be receptive. If there is no reponse, further investigation should be made before starting treatment.

Induction of ovulation using anti-oestrogens

If bleeding does occur after the progesterone challenge, then the anti-oestrogen clomiphene, 50mg once a day for five days, is usually the drug of first choice. Treatment is recommended early in the cycle, e.g. day two to day six, as there is evidence of decreased penetrability of cervical mucus to sperm during this stage of the cycle. This therapy can also be given later, from day six to day ten inclusively. Serum progesterone levels are checked in the luteal phase and, if they are still low, clomiphene should be increased to a maximum of 150mg daily. Cyclofenil or tamoxifen are alternative oral preparations. Side-effects are rare and relatively trivial, including hot flushes, nausea and frequency of micturition. The conception rate is approximately 50 per cent with an increased incidence of multiple births (particularly twins), and the patient should be made fully aware of this. The incidence of abortion and congenital anomalies in pregnancy after treatment is controversial. The increased incidence probably reflects the increased age of the patients as well as decreased fertility potential. Ovarian hyperstimulation with oral treatment is very rare and resolves on cessation of treatment, but a regular pelvic examination to check on ovarian size is recommended, particularly after any increase in dosage.

Induction of ovulation using gonadotrophins

Gonadotrophin preparations are expensive and potentially hazardous, as they can cause hyperstimulation (see below), and should only be prescribed when there are clear indications for their use, such as anovulation unresponsive to anti-oestrogens. The most commonly used preparation is human menopausal gonadotrophin extracted from human menopausal urine. It contains FSH and LH, although FSH action predominates, and it is marketed as Pergonal. Metrodin is a similar preparation with a lower LH response, leading to a more favourable LH:FSH ratio.

Treatment cycle
The theoretical basis of treatment is relatively simple, giving Pergonal or Metrodin to mature the follicles and then inducing ovulation with HCG which causes an LH surge. In fact, management is complicated and expensive, involving patient time, laboratory investigations and drug expense. This is illustrated in Fig. 8.2.
  (i) Mensturation occurs either naturally or following progesterone adminstration. Day one is the first day.
  (ii) FSH/LH is commenced on day six or day seven.
  (iii) Urinary (or blood) oestrogen levels are measured and ultrasound is performed to assess follicular size.

143

(iv) Repeated doses of FSH/LH are given on alternate days or occasionally on a daily basis until oestrogen levels have reached their target or follicles are the appropriate size (Fig. 8.2).

(v) HCG 10 000 IU is given intramuscularly to trigger ovulation.

(vi) Sexual intercourse must take place at least once in the next 48 hours.

(vii) If pregnancy does not occur the cycle is repeated, increasing the dose of FSH as indicated by oestrogen levels. If there is an excessive ovarian response, treatment is ceased and the patient advised to use barrier contraception because of the risk of multiple pregnancy. Often four-six months of treatment are required to achieve pregnancy, but long-term therapy is not indicated.

Use of LH-RH Analogues

Inhibitory effect (down regulation)

Luteinizing hormone releasing hormone (LH-RH) provokes secretion of luteinizing hormone (LH) and follicle stimulating hormone (FSH) by the anterior pituitary. Repeated administration of LH-RH agonists initially stimulate and then desensitize the pituitary cells responsible for producing gonado-trophins (LH and FSH). The continuous exposure of LH-RH receptors to LH-RH causes 'down-regulation' and in effect a medical hypophysectomy is created. If, however, LH-RH is administered in a pulsatile fashion (thereby stimulating normal LH-RH secretion) it will have a stimulatory effect. There are two therapeutic roles for LH-RH in infertility which depend upon the mode of administration.

First there may be a role for continuous administration in the treatment of women who have had unsuccessful ovulation induction attempts with clomiphene and exogenous gonadotrophins (hMG). The agonist is administered in the midluteal phase for ten to 14 days and a hypothalamic hypogonadal state confirmed. Thereafter daily gonadotrophin (Pergonal or Metrodin) injections are administered. Following a satisfactory rise in serum oestradiol associated with development of ovarian follicles, ovulation is induced with hCG and LH-RH agonist treatment is discontinued. Luteal phase support of the endometrium is provided by hCG injections or progesterone supplements. This treatment is, however, only appropriate under close medical supervision as there is a risk of multiple pregnancy

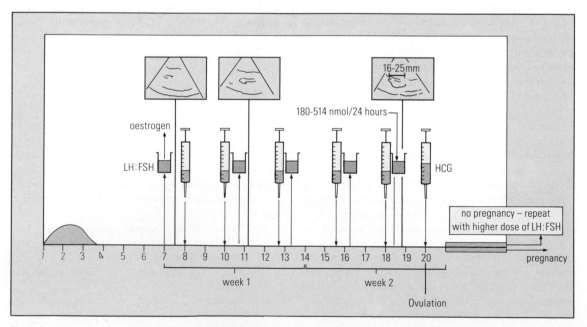

Fig. 8.2   Induction of ovulation using gonadotrophin.

and hyperstimulation. It is usually reserved for assisted reproduction programmes.

Stimulatory effect

An indication for utilizing the stimulatory action of LH-RH is ovulation induction when the preparation is administered in a pulsatile manner, either subcutaneously or intravenously. Administration in this manner would be appropriate for the patient with LH-RH deficiency or impairment. Such conditions may include weight-, stress-, and exercise- related amenorrhoea, and following surgery, trauma, and irrigation of the hypothalamic and pituitary areas.

Hyperstimulation

Complications of hyperstimulation may be very serious. The patient and her husband must be aware of the potential risks before embarking on treatment. Multiple pregnancies occur in between 12 and 45 per cent of pregnancies, depending on the degree of control. Most are twin pregnancies, but bigger multiples are seen and may suggest poor management. Obviously there is an increase in maternal and fetal complications with multiple pregnancies.

Mild hyperstimulation

Mild hyperstimulation occurs in approximately six per cent of cases. There is ovarian enlargement with some abdominal pain, but no specific treatment is required.

Moderate hyperstimulation

A moderate level of hyperstimulation results in a detectable, but not large, ovarian cyst. Abdominal pain, nausea and diarrhoea are common symptoms, but rest and symptomatic treatment is sufficient.

Severe hyperstimulation

Severe cases occur in approximately two per cent of treatments and can be life-threatening in a previously healthy woman. They present with severe abdominal pain caused by large ovarian cysts and ascites. Ovarian necrosis and intraperitoneal heamorrhage may occur. Hydrothorax has also been seen and can cause respiratory embarrassment. Because of the ascites, haemoconcentration occurs to the extent that it may cause arterial thrombosis. Management is as conservative as possible, with hospitalization, bed rest and intravenous fluids. Peritoneal drainage of ascites is frequently required and all this fluid loss must be replaced with protein-rich fluids. Careful electrolyte balance is important. Laparotomy is only required if the cysts rupture or there is intraperitoneal bleeding.

Summary

Induction of ovulation is an expensive and time-consuming procedure. Patients with hyperprolactinaemia usually respond well to bromocriptine (with or without the addition of clomiphene), which is simple and relatively inexpensive. Patients who have anovulation due to polycystic ovarian disease, where there is excessive androgen production suppressing follicular development, respond well to anti-oestrogens. Hypothalamic pituitary dysfunction may be resistant to treatment with anti-oestrogens in which case gonadotrophin therapy is used, which is more expensive and often results in other complications

CONTRACEPTION

The use of oestrogen and progesterones in the prevention of pregnancy is discussed in chapter nine.

CONTROL OF MENSTRUAL SYMPTOMS

Progesterones are particularly useful for helping to control menstrual flow, regulate the cycle and reduce premenstrual tension. They are frequently used in women with dysfunctional uterine bleeding (see chapter four). More recently, danazol has been used for similar problems, particularly to stop menstruation completely in patients with endometriosis, where a pseudopregnancy state is created (see chapter five).

HORMONE REPLACEMENT THERAPY (HRT)

The symptoms associated with the menopause may be minor or severe (Fig. 8.3). At this time in a woman's life her natural production of hormones (particularly oestrogen and progesterone) fall, and HRT acts to replace these and to prevent the symptoms and signs associated with the menopause (Fig. 8.4 and 8.5). Osteoporosis is a serious consequence of decreased oestrogen production which results in calcium loss from the bone at approximately one per cent per year. Eventually, substantial bone loss occurs so that fractures occur easily. One in four women over 60 years of age will suffer an osteoporosis-related fracture of some sort, increasing to one in two over the age of 70 years.

Although there is substantial evidence to prove that HRT halts this bone loss in menopausal women, there are a number of factors to be considered.

(i) Treatment must begin early because, once the bones are thin, introduction of therapy will merely prevent further loss, and not strengthen the existing weak bones.

(ii) Evidence suggests that once HRT is stopped there is rapid loss of calcium so that eventually there is little difference between those patients treated and those not. Therefore, for long-lasting results, HRT is required for the rest of the woman's life.

(iii) Cost is a major factor in preventing widespread and long-term use of HRT. The cost must be weighed against the potential benefits of reduced fractures in old women, which result in long hospital stays. The physical and psychological 'cost' must also be borne in mind.

(iv) Continuing menstruation into the seventies may be unacceptable to some women; hence HRT is predominantly used for relatively short-term therapy at the time of the menopause, and only used for long-term therapy in patients at particular risk of developing osteoporosis.

Most menopausal women have mild symptoms and so do not require regular HRT. Topical oestrogen creams can be used when patients complain of vaginal dryness, soreness or recurrent vaginal infections. Even in mild cases of prolapse, oestrogen creams may improve skin turgor and, in combination with pelvic floor exercises, may improve any urinary problems. Care must be taken to monitor the use of creams since appreciable systemic levels can be achieved, and it is important to know how often oestrogens are being used, and follow up appropriately. Progesterones alone may be used in patients with contra-indications to oestrogen therapy, e.g. endometrial carcinoma, and, if used in doses appropriate for menopausal women, may help to decrease anxiety and improve the patient's feeling of well-being. Medroxyprogesterone acetate 5-10mg once a day will suppress menopausal flushes in most cases.

Contraindications to HRT

When assessing which women to treat, certain contra-indications must be borne in mind. HRT should be used primarily to treat actual disease, the exception being potential osteoporosis. Therefore,

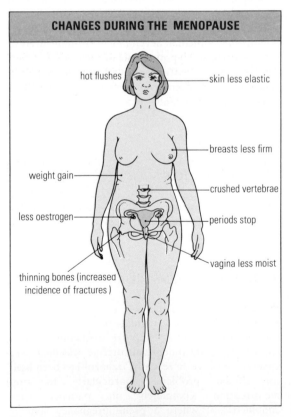

CHANGES DURING THE MENOPAUSE

hot flushes
skin less elastic
breasts less firm
weight gain
crushed vertebrae
less oestrogen
periods stop
vagina less moist
thinning bones (increased incidence of fractures)

Fig. 8.3 Changes during the menopause.

certain groups of women should not use this therapy at all. In particular, patients with the following:

(i) History of thromboembolism.

(ii) Oestrogen-dependent tumours e.g. breast or endometrium.

(iii) Liver disease, e.g. chronic hepatitis or cirrhosis.

(iv) Pre-existing coronary artery disease.

(v) Porphyria.

(vi) Hyperlipidaemia.

Careful consideration of the benefits must be made in women who are obese, hypertensive, diabetic, heavy smokers or who have varicose veins.

Beneficial effects of HRT

Similarly, there are groups of women in whom HRT may be particularly beneficial. It is important that doctors identify such women, and offer HRT at an early age postmenopausally, or perimenopausally.

(i) Inactive women who have an increased risk of osteoporosis (Fig. 8.6).

(ii) Women who have had previous fractures because of osteoporosis, and women with a strong family history of the condition.

(iii) Women who undergo premature menopause have been found to have an increased incidence of cardiovascular disease because of their diminished oestrogen levels.

(vi) Patients with type II lipoproteinaemia.

Side effects of HRT (Fig. 8.7)

Bleeding

Postmenopausal women may not welcome the return of regular withdrawal bleeds. Irregular or unexpected bleeding must be investigated.

Increased cancer risk

Endometrial hyperplasia and endometrial carcinoma are known to be increased in women who take unopposed oestrogen therapy (Figs. 8.8 and 8.9). The risk of endocervical carcinoma is up to five times greater in these women. Therapy in those who have a uterus should therefore include at least seven days of progesterone to cause a withdrawal bleed, and so prevent this problem.

Breast changes

Breast changes can occur, particularly breast tenderness and sometimes mastitis. If this is a problem, consideration must be given to stopping therapy or using progesterone alone. There is no clear evidence that HRT increases the risk of breast carcinoma, although unopposed oestrogen therapy theoretically would increase the risk in oestrogen-receptor positive patients.

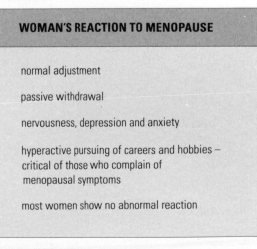

MENOPAUSE; WOMAN'S VIEW OF COMMON SYMPTOMS
depression
faulty memory
excessive weight gain
painful intercourse
brittle bones

Fig. 8.4 Menopause – woman's view of common symptoms.

WOMAN'S REACTION TO MENOPAUSE
normal adjustment
passive withdrawal
nervousness, depression and anxiety
hyperactive pursuing of careers and hobbies – critical of those who complain of menopausal symptoms
most women show no abnormal reaction

Fig. 8.5 Woman's reaction to menopause.

Thromboembolism
The incidence of thromboembolism may be increased further in those already at risk, and they should not take HRT. The risk of stroke or myocardial infarction has not been shown to be increased.

Diabetes
Diabetic control may be hindered, and a balanced decision regarding the necessity of treatment should be made. There are other minor side-effects.

Management

Patients requesting HRT need a careful history and examination to determine their risk factors and the potential benefits for them. The presence or absence of the uterus and ovaries is important in deciding on appropriate therapy. The patient's attitude to regular withdrawal bleeding should also be considered. Some of the processes involved in determining how to treat a woman with menopausal symptoms are summarized in Fig. 8.10. The benefits and side-effects of treatment should also be fully discussed (Fig. 8.11).

Unopposed oestrogens
Unopposed oestrogens can be used as: (1) oral preparations; (2) an implant; or (3) a transdermal patch. These should be prescribed only for patients who have had a hysterectomy, because the use of unopposed oestrogens increases the risk of developing endometrial carcinoma. This significantly increased risk of endometrial cancer in women with an intact uterus is not acceptable in today's

FACTORS ASSOCIATED WITH AN INCREASED RISK OF POSTMENOPAUSAL OSTEOPOROSIS

premature menopause

Caucasian race

small build

nulliparity

sedentary life-style

alcohol abuse

cigarette smoking

high caffeine intake

corticosteroid therapy

high protein diet

Fig. 8.6 Factors associated with an increased risk of postmenopausal osteoporosis.

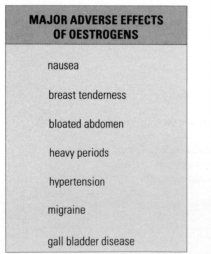

MAJOR ADVERSE EFFECTS OF OESTROGENS

nausea

breast tenderness

bloated abdomen

heavy periods

hypertension

migraine

gall bladder disease

Fig. 8.7 Adverse effects of oestrogens.

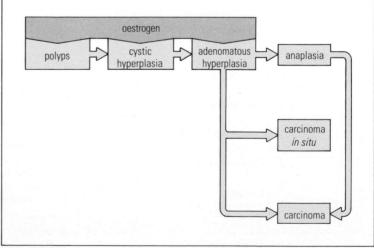

Fig. 8.8 Histogenesis of endometrial carcinoma.

gynaecological practice, even if regular uterine curettage is performed.

Combined oestrogen and progesterone

Cyclical oestrogen and progesterone therapy producing regular withdrawal bleeding should be used in women who still have a uterus, during and after the menopause. There are several oral preparations marketed in calendar packs. Alternatively, oestrogens may be given by implant or skin patch with seven to ten days of oral progesterone each month. It is hoped that a combined oestrogen and progesterone transdermal patch may be available in the future. The drawbacks of implants are that they usually last for six months and tend to given high peak doses with an uncertain duration of action, and, once administered, the dose cannot be altered. They also require a small skin incision for insertion on each occasion. They have become less popular.

In choosing a preparation it is important to consider the following principles:

(i) Use the minimum dose to relieve symptoms effectively or provide necessary prophylaxis.
(ii) Adjust the dose regime to suit the patient.
(iii) Adjust the duration of therapy to suit the patient.

All patients on HRT need regular follow up at approximately six month intervals, including regular blood pressure checks, vaginal examinations and a record of their bleeding.

Miscellaneous conditions

Topical oestrogen use has been mentioned above in connection with the menopause. Local oestrogen creams may also be used to decrease vulval irritation and improve the quality of smear-taking in older women in whom smear follow-up is important. Testosterone creams are occasionally used for pruritus vulvae, but great care must be taken because of the virilizing properties. Oestrogen is used to develop secondary sexual characteristics in conditions such as Turner's syndrome. Progesterone may be used preoperatively to decrease bleeding in

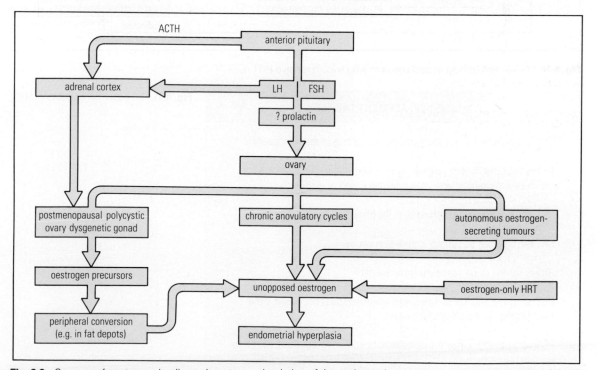

Fig. 8.9 Sources of oestrogen leading to long-term stimulation of the endometrium unopposed by progesterone.

endometrial carcinoma and postoperatively to prevent recurrence of the tumour; it may also be used in those unfit for surgery. There is no real evidence to substantiate the use of any hormones in maintaining early pregnancy. Although the administration of HCG may be useful, the real success of the treatment is almost certainly a combination of a placebo effect and additional care given to those women with recurrent abortions.

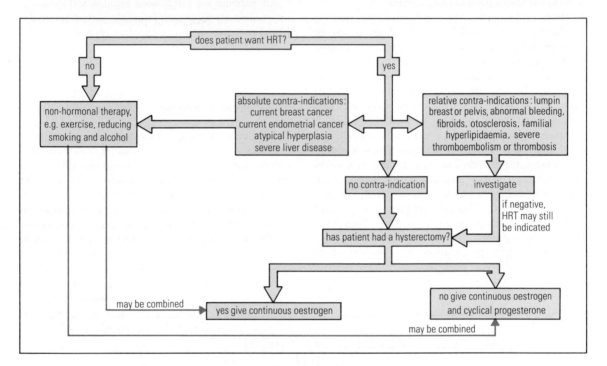

Fig. 8.10 Flow chart to help in decision as to who should receive HRT.

Fig. 8.11 The potential benefits of HRT.

HORMONE REPLACEMENT THERAPY

HRT replaces the natural hormones that are lacking at the menopause

HRT relieves hot flushes, vaginal dryness, frequent urination and other unpleasant symptoms, when these are due to lack of oestrogen

HRT also helps to prevent thinning of the bones

HRT can be taken as tablets, creams or implants

HRT is not the same as the contraceptive pill

HRT using combined oestrogen and progestogen does not increase the risk of cancer of the lining of the womb

HRT occasionally causes breast tenderness or nausea, but these can often be cured by changing to a different type of preparation

9   Contraception and Sterilization

INTRODUCTION

There are many methods of birth control of varying popularity of use. The increasing occurrence of sexually transmitted diseases, including AIDS, has lead to an increased use of barrier methods which help prevent the spread of infection. Similarly, with improved infant mortality rates and smaller family sizes the demand for sterilization has increased (both male and female), particularly in younger couples. Adverse press articles on 'the pill' can lead to a temporary reduction in its use and, unfortunately, this is often followed by a rise in unwanted pregnancies. This chapter describes the different methods of contraception and sterilization available and discusses their effectiveness, safety and convenience of use.

CONTRACEPTION

Contraception is used for the temporary prevention of pregnancy for personal, social, medical or genetic reasons. When discussing contraception, a careful history needs to be taken, particularly to discover contraindications for any particular method, e.g. deep vein thrombosis (DVT) for the combined pill, or a history of pelvic inflammatory disease for the IUCD. Consideration should also be given to the patient's age, intelligence and lifestyle. General examination must include blood pressure and weight, and a pelvic examination is appropriate in all women including a cervical smear.

Contraception can be divided into three main groups:
(i) Natural;
(ii) Mechanical;
(iii) Hormonal.

Natural methods of contraception

Coitus interruptus

Coitus interruptus is the oldest and probably still the most widely used method of contraception. It is moderately effective, simple and medically safe. It involves removal of the penis from the vagina before ejaculation occurs. Failure occurs from delay in withdrawal, or because the pre-ejaculatory fluid may contain some spermatozoa.

'Safe period' methods

There are various methods of predicting the fertile and infertile phases in the cycle and a combination of these is frequently used (illustrated in Fig. 9.1).

Cyclical temperature changes

Cyclical temperature changes at ovulation may be determined by taking the basal body temperature, usually per vaginum or rectum immediately upon wakening. Twenty-four to thirty-six hours prior to ovulation there is a temperature drop and then there is a rise of 0.4°C one to two days after ovulation, thereafter remaining at a plateau. The couple abstain from sexual intercourse until three days after the temperature rise. Great accuracy of temperature record and motivation are required.

Rhythm or calender method

With this technique sexual intercourse should be avoided between 18 to 11 days before the next period is due to avoid the fertile phase. Women need to define the shortest and longest menstrual cycles over the previous 12 cycles. For those with irregular cycles or following childbirth the potential fertile phase may be unacceptably long.

Changes in cervical mucus

Cervical mucus changes may be useful as an indicator because mucus becomes profuse and watery at ovulation. Women can be taught to recognise these changes as well as changes in the cervix itself, which becomes softer and 'gaping' at ovulation.

Although natural family planning is becoming increasingly popular, it does have a high failure rate even in well motivated couples at 15%. It is acceptable to religious groups, e.g. Catholics, but to be effective requires regular menstrual cycles and limits sexual intercourse to only short periods during the cycle.

Prolongation of lactation
Women are less fertile when breast feeding and this method of spacing children has long been used,

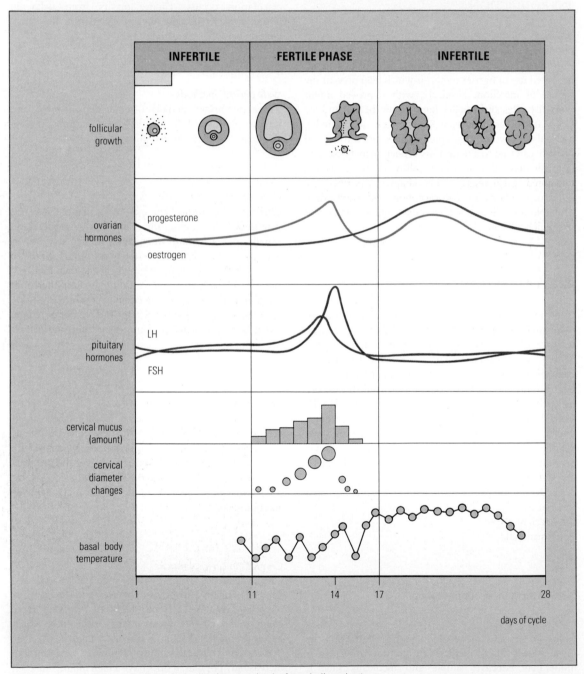

Fig. 9.1 Prediction of the fertile and infertile phases using 'safe period' methods.

particularly in the developing world. However, the suppression of ovulation during lactation is very variable and it is not a very effective method in a well nourished population.

Mechanical methods of contraception

The various mechanical forms of contraception are listed in Fig. 9.2, those most commonly used are the sheath, diaphragm and IUCD (coil). The first two are commonly known as barrier methods. Cervical caps, contraceptive

sponges and female condoms are available, although less commonly used. Often spermicides are used in conjunction e.g. with the condom, although they may also be used alone.

Condoms
The condom, or sheath, is the only form of contraception presently available which can be used by the man. It is a closed and tubally designed device to cover the erect penis and prevent transmission of semen into the vagina. Most are made of thin vulcanized rubber and may be lubricated. Condoms may be accused of decreasing sensitivity, but also help to prevent the spread of sexually transmitted diseases. They are easily obtainable and can be used with spermicides for extra protection.

A female condom has been produced (see Fig. 9.4), but it is not yet widely available. It is aimed particularly at women with multiple partners.

Diaphragm
The diaphragm (cap) consists of a thin latex rubber hemisphere with a flexible metal spring made in a range of sizes. It fits across the cervix as shown in Fig. 9.3. The

MECHANICAL METHODS OF CONTRACEPTION	
condom (sheath)	
diaphragm (cap)	barrier
contraceptive sponge	methods
female condom	
intraterine contraceptive device (IUCD or coil)	
spermicides	

Fig. 9.2 Mechanical forms of contraception.

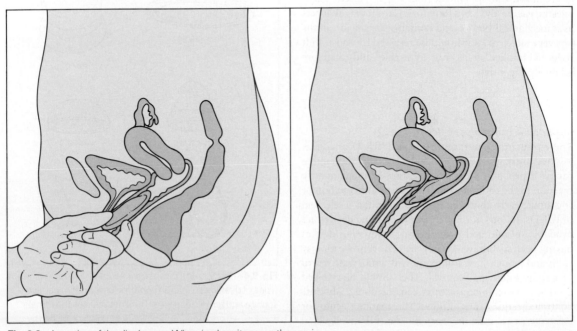

Fig. 9.3 Insertion of the diaphragm. When in place it covers the cervix.

cap prevents sperm from getting to the cervix and because it is left in place for 6 to 12 hours after intercourse, most sperm are killed by the acidity of the vagina. A spermicide, applied around the rim, or as a pessary, is advised, particularly for repeated sexual intercourse. After use it is washed with soap and water and stored.

When assessing the size of diaphragm required a careful pelvic examination is required. The distance between the posterior fornix and symphysis pubis should be estimated and an appropriate size diaphragm (in millimetres) of the same diameter chosen.

Women need careful fitting and guidance in the use of the cap. It is essential that they can demonstrate the correct insertion and removal. Re-assessment of size is required after childbirth or following weight increase or decrease. Its efficacy is comparable to the sheath, but some consider it 'messy' and its use had fallen until a recent revival in view of its 'barrier' nature.

Others types of cap include the cervical cap which fits the cervix closely and vault cap which stays in place by suction, although not in contact with the cervix (Fig. 9.4).

Contraceptive sponge

The contraceptive sponge is made of polyurethane foam impregnated with spermicide (Fig. 9.4). It is inserted high into the vagina and has a loop for ease of removal. It acts as a mechanical barrier and contains spermicide, but is not very effective and should be reserved for those with reduced fertility. It is not re-usable and therefore relatively expensive.

Intrauterine contraceptive device (IUCD)

The intrauterine contraceptive device (IUCD or coil) is inserted through the cervix and placed in the uterine cavity. It probably works by creating an inflammatory reaction in the endometrium to prevent implantation or encourage early abortion. Fig. 9.5 illustrates a selection of IUCDs. In the UK only copper containing devices are available (plastic and progesterone containing devices having been withdrawn). They are relatively cheap, easy to fit and require little follow up with immediate return of fertility following removal. They should be changed every 4–5 years (manufacturer's instructions). Absolute contraindications are known pregnancy, acute or subacute pelvic inflammatory disease (PID), congenital uterine anomalies, abnormal uterine bleeding of un-

known cause, valvular heart disease or carcinoma of the cervix or endometrium.

The IUCD can be used as a form of post-coital contraception by inserting it up to five days after the calculated ovulation date. It works by preventing implantation of the fertilized ovum.

Insertion

Insertion is best carried out during menstruation or shortly after as the cervix is slightly open, having carefully examined for size, shape and mobility of the uterus. Aseptic technique should be employed. The uterus is sounded for length, the trocar length adjusted appropriately and then the IUCD inserted into the uterine cavity through the cervix until the fundus is reached. The trocar is removed leaving the IUCD behind and the thread trimmed (Fig. 9.6). The thread is for removal at a later date. Appropriate training in the insertion of an IUCD is needed to reduce the risk of perforation of the uterus at insertion.

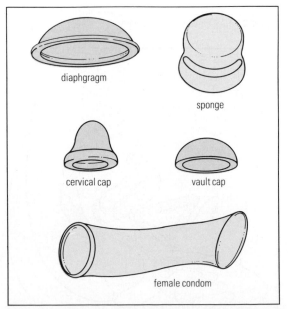
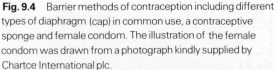

diaphgragm

sponge

cervical cap

vault cap

female condom

Fig. 9.4 Barrier methods of contraception including different types of diaphragm (cap) in common use, a contraceptive sponge and female condom. The illustration of the female condom was drawn from a photograph kindly supplied by Chartce International plc.

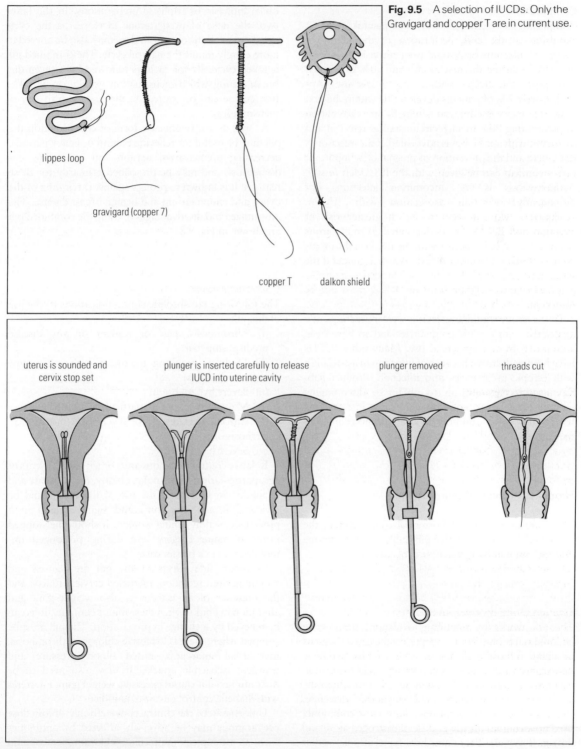

Fig. 9.5 A selection of IUCDs. Only the Gravigard and copper T are in current use.

lippes loop

gravigard (copper 7)

copper T

dalkon shield

uterus is sounded and cervix stop set

plunger is inserted carefully to release IUCD into uterine cavity

plunger removed

threads cut

Fig. 9.6 Insertion of an IUCD.

155

Complications

Complications include heavy or painful periods, expulsion of the coil, perforation of the uterus at insertion, infection or ectopic pregnancy. Expulsion is most likely during the first month and 10% of women will expel the IUCD within one year's use. Approximately 2% of patients develop PID within the first year, although some infections may be an exacerbation of pre-existing PID. In such circumstances removal and treatment with antibiotics is advocated. If the infection is not severe and the prevention of pregnancy is important then treatment can be given with the IUCD left *in situ*. Actinomycosis is an uncommon infection, not infrequently seen in association with IUCDs. Nulliparous women seem to be at greater risk of infection and IUCDs are better suited to multiparous women. If pregnancy occurs with the IUCD in the uterus there is a high rate of miscarriage, which is greater if the IUCD is not removed. The increased incidence of ectopic pregnancy in association with the IUCD must not be forgotten.

Progesterone containing devices were more frequently associated with ectopic pregnancies and so have been withdrawn from commercial use. Many other IUCDs have been withdrawn because of litigation in association with ectopic pregnancies and infection. Product liability insurance is difficult to obtain so discouraging manufacturers from continuing research and making IUCDs. It is possible they may become a contraception of the past.

Hormonal methods of contraception

There are three types of hormonal contraception, the combined oral contraceptive pill (pill), the progesterone only pill (mini pill), or injectible progesterone.

Combined oral contraceptive pill

The pill works by inhibiting ovulation, suppressing endometrial proliferation and altering the cervical mucus to make it hostile to sperm. One of two synthetic oestrogens are in use, ethinyl oestradiol and mestranol. The most widely used progesterones are norethisterone, levonorgestrol, lynestrenol and ethynodiol diacetate. There are various preparations, those most commonly used now contain the lower dose of oestrogen at 30 and 35 μg, (Fig. 9.7). There are three types of pill – either those where the pill is exactly the same throughout the

cycle, biphasic or triphasic preparations. In the latter two, the dose of progesterone increases as the cycle progresses and the oestrogen dose may also be altered to more closely mimic the natural cycle. The combined pill is taken cyclically for 21 days followed by a seven day break during which menstruation usually occurs. The first course can be started on the first or fifth day of menstruation.

As well as a very effective form of contraception the pill may be useful for relieving painful or heavy periods, decreasing premenstrual tension and controlling endometriosis and may be prescribed primarily for these reasons. It is known to protect against carcinoma of the ovary and endometrium and benign breast disease. The advantages and disadvantages of using the combined pill are shown in Fig. 9.8.

Contraindications

The following are absolute contraindications to the use of the pill:

(i) Thrombosis, past or present or any disease predisposing to it;

(ii) Migraine requiring treatment with ergotamine containing drugs;

(iii) Severe hypertension;

(iv) Malignant neoplasm, particularly of the breast;

(v) Chronic liver disease or severe liver disease, e.g. cirrhosis or porphyrias;

(vi) Severe heart disease.

Relative contraindications are women over 35 years of age, particularly if they smoke, obesity, renal disease and cholilithiasis. Obviously the use of the pill should be reviewed if any symptoms and signs develop in a previously healthy young woman. It should be stopped prior to major surgery and during prolonged immobilization in a plaster cast.

Common side effects of the pill are nausea and vomiting, fluid retention, increased cervical mucus and the presence of an ectropion, also weight gain and alteration in libido. Often these minor complications can be relieved by a change in preparation. The pill must be stopped where there is extensive chloasma, thrombosis, myocardial infarction, raised blood pressure and transient ischaemic attacks. It may also need to be discontinued if it causes excessive weight gain, interferes with diabetic control or causes jaundice.

Unfortunately, the contraceptive efficacy of low dose preparations may be adversely affected by antibiotics such as rifampicin, ampicillin, chloramphenicol and neomycin. Due to liver enzyme induction epileptics on

CURRENTLY AVAILABLE CONTRACEPTIVE PILLS

Pill type	Preparation	Oestrogen (μg)	Progestogen (μg)
Combined *Ethinyloestradiol/ norethisterone type*	Loestrin 20	20	1
	Loestrin 30	30	1.5
	Conova 30	30	2
	Brevinor	35	0.5
	Ovysmen	35	0.5
	Neocon 1/35	35	1
	Norimin	35	1
	Minilyn	50	2.5
Ethinyloestradiol/ levonorgestrel	Microgynon 30	30	0.15
	Ovranette	30	0.15
	Eugynon 30	30	0.25
	Ovran 30	30	0.25
	Ovran	50	0.25
Ethinyloestradiol/ desogestrel	Mercilon	20	0.15
	Marvelon	30	0.15
Ethinyloestradiol/ gestodene	Femodene	30	0.075
	Minulet	30	0.075
Mestranol/ norethisterone	Norinyl-1	50	1
	Ortho-Novin 1/50	50	1

Pill type	Preparation	Oestrogen (μg)	Progestogen (μg)
Biphasic & Triphasic *Ethinyloestradiol/ norethisterone*	Binovum	35 / 35	0.5 / 1
	Synphase	35 / 35	0.5 / 1
	Trinovum	35 / 35 / 35	0.5 / 0.75 / 1
Ethinyloestradiol/ levonorgestrel	Logynon (also ED)	30 / 40 / 30	0.05 / 0.075 / 0.125
	Trinordiol	30 / 40 / 30	0.05 / 0.075 / 0.125
Progestogen only *Norethisterone type*	Micronor	–	0.35
	Noriday	–	0.35
	Femulen	–	0.5
Levonorgestrel	Microval	–	0.03
	Norgeston	–	0.03
	Neogest	–	0.075

Fig. 9.7 List of currently available contraceptive pills.

157

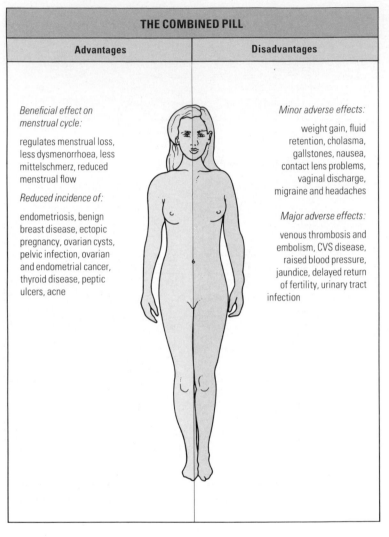

THE COMBINED PILL	
Advantages	**Disadvantages**
Beneficial effect on menstrual cycle: regulates menstrual loss, less dysmenorrhoea, less mittelschmerz, reduced menstrual flow *Reduced incidence of:* endometriosis, benign breast disease, ectopic pregnancy, ovarian cysts, pelvic infection, ovarian and endometrial cancer, thyroid disease, peptic ulcers, acne	*Minor adverse effects:* weight gain, fluid retention, cholasma, gallstones, nausea, contact lens problems, vaginal discharge, migraine and headaches *Major adverse effects:* venous thrombosis and embolism, CVS disease, raised blood pressure, jaundice, delayed return of fertility, urinary tract infection

Fig. 9.8 Advantages and disadvantages of using the combined pill.

phenobarbitone or phenytoin need a higher oestrogen dose pill. Oral contraceptives potentiate the effect of oral anticoagulants, although such women should not be on the pill.

Progesterone only pill

The progesterone only pill contains no oestrogen and consists of a small daily dose of progesterone. They are thought to work by changing the endometrium to make it unresponsive to implantation and by altering the cervical mucus, rendering it hostile to sperm. They are also thought to decrease tubal motility and cause incomplete ovulation suppression.

They are less effective than the combined pill, may result in irregular menstruation, but are free from oestrogen induced side effects such as the increased risk of thrombo-embolic disease. Progesterone only pills do not inhibit lactation and are therefore very useful for breastfeeding mothers and may be used in patients who are older, smoke or have a history of thrombosis or liver disease.

Contraindications

There are no absolute contraindications, but relative ones include:

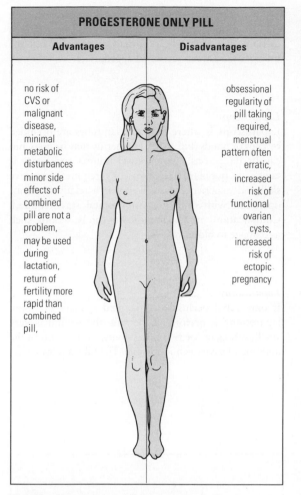

PROGESTERONE ONLY PILL	
Advantages	Disadvantages
no risk of CVS or malignant disease, minimal metabolic disturbances minor side effects of combined pill are not a problem, may be used during lactation, return of fertility more rapid than combined pill,	obsessional regularity of pill taking required, menstrual pattern often erratic, increased risk of functional ovarian cysts, increased risk of ectopic pregnancy

Fig. 9.9 Advantages and disadvantages of using the progesterone only pill.

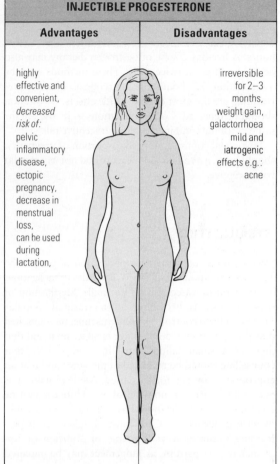

INJECTIBLE PROGESTERONE	
Advantages	Disadvantages
highly effective and convenient, *decreased risk of:* pelvic inflammatory disease, ectopic pregnancy, decrease in menstrual loss, can be used during lactation,	irreversible for 2–3 months, weight gain, galactorrhoea mild and **iatrogenic** effects e.g.: acne

Fig. 9.10 Advantages and disadvantages of using injectible progesterone

(i) Menstrual irregularity, as it may confuse the diagnosis;
(ii) A higher risk of ectopic pregnancies;
(iii) After a hydatidiform mole until the urine is clear of HCG;
(iv) In malabsorption syndrome of the gastrointestinal system;
(v) Severe liver disorders with persistent biochemical change.

For the progesterone only pill to be an effective form of contraception it must be taken at the same time each day and this regularity is an important part of its efficacy. Other advantages and disadvantages of this type of pill are listed in Fig. 9.9.

Injectible preparations
Depo preparations, most commonly using 150mg medroxy progesterone acetate, may be given at three monthly intervals. They work by inhibition of ovulation at the hypothalamic level with abolition of cyclic LH/FSH and oestradiol secretions. There are also contraceptive effects on luteal and tubal function, endometrium and cervical mucus. Menstruation tends to be irregular and may be prolonged and heavy. Amenorrhoea occurs in about 30% of women within one year of use. Fig. 9.10 lists the main advantages and disadvantages in the use of injectibles. Menstrual cycles and fertility usually return to normal six months after the last injection.

159

Post-coital (commonly called 'morning after') pill

The commonly used method is to use 100μg ethinyl oestradiol and 500μg levonorgestrol (e.g. 2 × Ovran 50 tablets) given immediately and repeated after twelve hours. A five-day course of oestrogen therapy may also be used and given twice daily. These methods must be used within 72 hours of intercourse. Nausea and vomiting are the most common side effects. Medication should be repeated. Contraindications to its use are the same as for the combined oral contraceptive pill.

Post-coital contraception, like abortion of pregnancy, should be seen as a first aid measure and not as a regular contraceptive.

STERILIZATION

Sterilization is the permanent prevention of pregnancy. The most commonly performed method is tubal ligation/ interruption or vasectomy in the male. Sterilization of either partner is becoming an increasingly popular method of birth control. The patients must be counselled that the operation is deemed irreversible, final and that there is a small failure rate. It is imperative that counselling should be recorded in the notes and that an appropriate consent form is used. Medicolegally it is essential to warn that no surgical procedure can ever be guaranteed and sterilizations have been a common cause of alleged negligence. Care must be taken when performing sterilization at the time of abortion or immediately post partum, as judgement may be impaired by recent events.

Male sterilization

Male sterilization or vasectomy is a simple procedure which can be performed under local anaesthetic. It involves division and ligation of the vas deferens on each side (Fig. 9.11). Ejaculates must be free of sperm before sterility is assumed and this usually takes three months post-operation. It is related more to the number of post-operative ejaculations than time. At least two semen analyses should be examined and found negative.

Female sterilization

Female sterilization is usually performed by laparoscopy

or laparotomy. Hysterectomy may be the appropriate choice in a woman with other problems such as menorrhagia. Tubal ligation may be performed at the time of a Caesarean section, if appropriate.

Laparoscopy

Laparoscopy is where the Fallopian tubes are occluded by clips or bands (Fig. 9.12). Diathermy may be used, but can be dangerous due to bowel trauma and hence is falling in popularity. Laparoscopy requires operative skill and experience as well, but is a relatively minor operation with only a short hospital stay required. Complications are uncommon, but can be serious, such as damage to blood vessels.

Laparotomy

If only tubal occlusion is required a small or 'mini' laparotomy is performed. Because the wound is very small, sufficient for two fingers only, exploration of the abdominal cavity is not possible. The tube and ovary on

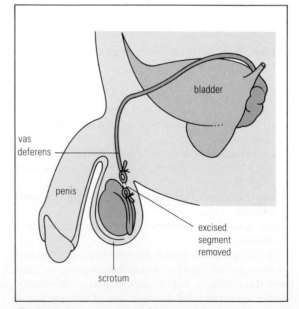

Fig. 9.11 Vasectomy procedure.

each side are delivered, the tube is divided and ligated and returned with the ovary to the abdomen. Histology confirms complete division of the Fallopian tube. There are various techniques with or without separation to the cut ends (Fig. 9.13).

Failures occur most commonly because the patient is unknowingly pregnant at the time of operation. Otherwise pregnancies usually occur within a year. Failures after this time are more rare and more likely to be ectopic pregnancies.

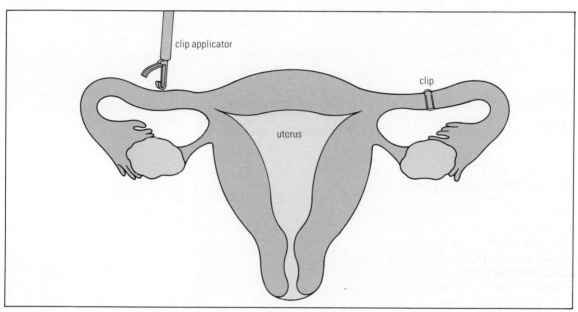

Fig. 9.12   Laparoscopic sterilization using clips.

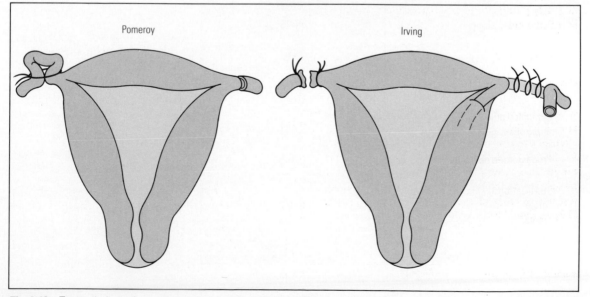

Fig. 9.13   Two techniques for surgical occlusion of the Fallopian tubes.

EFFECTIVENESS OF CONTRACEPTIVE METHODS

Contraceptive effectiveness is traditionally measured by means of the PEARL index which expresses failure in terms of numbers of pregnancies per 100 women years of exposure, i.e. the number of women who fall pregnant out of a group of 100 using a form of contraception for one year. User failure rates for the methods of contraception and sterilization discussed in this chapter are illustrated in Fig. 9.14.

The choice of contraception depends on the couple involved. Careful counselling is required to choose the appropriate method and a careful history to discover contraindications and lifestyles is important. In an age of increasing sexually transmitted disease, in particular AIDS, it is important to advise patients of all the risks of sexual intercourse.

FAILURE RATES FOR DIFFERENT METHODS OF CONTRACEPTION	
Method	**Range of failure/100 women years**

No method:
  young women
  age 40
  age 45
  age 50
	80–90
	40–60
	10–12
	0–5

Coitus interruptus	8–17
Natural family planning	6–25
Condom (male)	2–15
Spermicides alone	4–25
Diaphragm	2–15
IUCD	0.3–4
Combined pills 50 μg oestrogen	0.2–1
Progesterone only pill	0.3–5

Sterilization:
  male
  female
	0–0.2
	0–0.5

Fig. 9.14 Failure rates for different methods of contraception per 100 women years.

Principles of Radiotherapy and Chemotherapy

INTRODUCTION

Surgery, radiotherapy and chemotherapy are the three principal therapeutic modalities available for treatment of gynaecological malignancies. A considerable amount of experience has been gained as to what can and cannot be accomplished by each of these arms of treatment.

Some cancers, for example, which were previously considered incurable have been found to be curable by a combination of radiotherapy, chemotherapy and surgery. The best results, as judged by cure, occur when the decision as to the best treatment for an individual patient with gynaecological cancer is made by a multidisciplinary team approach rather than by a single specialist. It is also preferable for the various specialists to be involved at an early stage in the decision as to the most appropriate therapy for a particular patient. Unfortunately this does not happen often enough, to the detriment of the patient.

RADIATION THERAPY

The tools of radiation therapy are X-rays, gamma-rays, or energetic particles such as electrons, protons or neutrons. X-rays result from the rapid deceleration of fast moving electrons through a vacuum tube. Gamma-rays result from the variation in the energy state of an atom; these changes occur at a characteristic rate in atoms such as radium, cobalt, caesium and other radioactive isotopes. According to the power of penetration and source of the radiation, radiotherapy can be divided into four categories as shown in Fig. 10.1.

Radium used to be the most important radioactive isotope source of gamma radiation used for the treatment of carcinoma of the cervix and uterus. However, because of the inherent risk of radiation exposure to the staff treating the patient, it has been replaced in clinical practice by other isotopes, and in particular by caesium. Additionally, the use of after-loading devices for interstitial and intracavity treatment has further reduced the risks to staff.

The machines commonly used in the treatment of gynaecological cancers to generate X- or gamma-irradiation in the megavoltage range are the linear acceleration or telecobalt-60 machines. The advantages of megavoltage irradiation are:

(i)   Its skin sparing effect.
(ii) Its ability to deliver irradiation at a determined depth in the pelvis with minimal damage to adjacent normal organs or tissues.
(iii) Its bone sparing effect.
(iv) It produces less radiation sickness and is therefore better tolerated by the patient.

RADIOTHERAPEUTIC MODALITIES	
low voltage x-ray	50–120k used primarily for skin cancers
Kilovoltage x-ray	range is over several million volts, up to 25×10^6V and more; commonly used in treating gynaecological cancers
Megavoltage x-ray	200–400kV no place in gynaecological cancers
Gamma-ray sources of reletherapy	principally cobalt – 60 units.

Fig. 10.1 Four categories of radiotherapy, divided according to power of penetration.

163

When ionizing radiation irradiates cells and tissues, certain changes result. The radiation changes produce their effects on tumour and normal cells in a variety of ways by:

(i)   Metabolic changes.
(ii) Loss of reproductive ability.
(iii) Cell transformation.
(iv) Acceleration of cellular aging.
(v)   Mutation.

Injuries to individual cells may be to induce lethal damage, potentially lethal damage, or sublethal damage.

Tumours are extremely complex and variable in their make-up and some tumours respond better to radiotherapy than others. Clinically, radiosensitivity refers to gross tumour shrinkage. The classification of response to radiotherapy is somewhat arbitrary, but Fig. 10.2 indicates the response of certain gynaecological tumours.

Purpose of radiation therapy

The purpose of radiotherapy is threefold; for it to be either curative, palliative, or an adjunct to surgery.

Radical radiotherapy with the purpose of producing a cure is not without a certain amount of morbidity and should be carried out with care and justification. There can be both local and systemic radiation reactions, which are sometimes severe, but these have to be accepted in order to achieve cure.

The discomfort suffered by patients from curative radiation therapy is not less, and indeed is sometimes more, than that which follows radical surgery. If a patient is unsuitable for radical curative surgery due to a rapid deterioration in her condition for whatever reason, then she is equally unfit for curative radiotherapy.

When there is extensive disease which is incurable, then palliative radiotherapy for symptomatic relief may be appropriate. Symptoms such as pain, offensive discharge, ulceration or obstruction may be alleviated by a palliative dose of radiotherapy. The idea is to prolong a useful and comfortable life. Patients in the terminal phase of advanced malignancy and beyond palliative radiotherapy need kindness, comfort, analgesics such as Omnopon, and good nursing care.

Rationale for combined radiotherapy and surgery

Surgery and radiotherapy are equally effective in eradicating small limited cancers and each has its own merits, indications and limitations in treating gynaecological cancers. Radiotherapy has the advantage of being able to control the disease *in situ* and is therefore an organ-sparing procedure. Surgery for certain early lesions can, in many instances, be carried out without functional or cosmetic mutilation. Surgical failures are often related to the failure to remove microscopic tumour at the

RADIOSENSITIVITY OF GYNAECOLOGICAL TUMOURS
Very radiosensitive Dysgerminoma and granulosa cell tumours of the ovary
Radiosensitive Squamous cell carcinoma, adenocarcinoma and endometrioid carcinoma of the cervix and uterus
Epithelial ovarian tumours and oestrogen-induced clear cell carcinoma of the cervix and vagina
Relatively radioinsensitive Sarcomas, melanomas and ovarian malignant teratoma
Sarcoma botryoides

Fig. 10.2 Response to radiotherapy of some gynaecological tumours.

resection margin, whereas radiotherapy failures are often because it can fail to remove hypoxic cells at the centre of large tumours. Tumour seeding in the wound after surgery, and lymphatic and blood spread are additional reasons for surgical and radiotherapy failures.

The major role of radiotherapy is to eradicate the radiosensitive, actively growing, well-oxygenated cells in the periphery of a tumour; surgery is able to remove the centrally situated radioresistant hypoxic tumour cells. Therefore, for extensive tumours which are not curable by either surgery or radiotherapy alone, the logical approach is to combine therapy.

There is a place for preoperative radiotherapy in some cases of carcinoma of the cervix, and postoperative radiotherapy following surgery for carcinoma of the endometrium. It should be stressed that if radiotherapy is given preoperatively, a full dose of radiotherapy is not given, and so if the surgery is deferred or not carried out then the patient suffers because treatment has been inadequate. The aim of postoperative radiotherapy is to eradicate residual or subclinical disease at the operative site, e.g. vaginal vault after hysterectomy for carcinoma of the uterus.

Carcinoma of the cervix

Carcinoma of the cervix is the most common cancer of the female genital tract and in its early stages it is curable. Its radiotherapeutic control depends on the fact that the cervix and uterus have a high tolerance to radiation. In general they can stand a much higher dose of irradiation than other tissues in the body. For example, 7000-8000cGy can usually be delivered locally by intracavity caesium to the cervix, uterus and parametrium without significant radiation complications. This high dosage cannot be tolerated beyond 3-4cm lateral to the cervical canal; it is a localised treatment, and therefore a cancerocidal dose is not given to the entire parametrium and the pelvic side-walls. For advanced carcinomas, (stage IIB and stage III), the emphasis is on using external beam therapy as the treatment of choice followed by a reduced dosage of intracavity caesium. In general, a dose of 5500-6000cGy can be safely delivered to the lateral parametrium and pelvic wall lymph nodes by a combination of external beam irradiation and intracavity caesium.

The dosage of irradiation for carcinoma of the cervix is determined by the tolerance to the radiation of the rectum, rectovaginal septum, bladder and small bowel. The total dosage has to be reduced in women with pelvic inflammatory disease, in those with previous multiple pelvic and abdominal surgical operations, in women aged 70 and over, and in those who are in a physically debilitated condition.

Fig. 10.3 shows the three original principal methods of giving intracavity and vaginal radium, and explains their basic principle.

Since there is a high incidence of metastases in the pelvic nodes – of the order of 15 per cent in Stage I, 30 per cent in Stage II and 45 per cent in Stage III lesions – the management of carcinoma of the cervix must include treatment of both the primary lesion and the pelvic side-walls.

The role of surgery in the management of cancer of the cervix

Although radiotherapy is appropriate for most women with carcinoma of the cervix, there are some circumstances in which surgery may be preferred or be more appropriate, particularly for stages I and IIA. The preference will often depend on the experience and expertise of the surgeon, and knowledge of the radiotherapeutic facilities available. There is no doubt that the radiotherapist will always obtain better results than the occasional surgeon. The types of pathological conditions or radiotherapeutic problems which may indicate that surgical treatment is more appropriate are given in Fig. 10.4.

When there is central recurrence after full radiotherapy dosage, the possibility of surgery by some form of exenteration may have to be considered. This surgery should, however, be contemplated only when there is a reasonable chance of total cure. It is not a palliative procedure except in the presence of a urinary fistula.

Results of radiotherapy in carcinoma of the cervix

The results vary worldwide, but treatment of stage I carcinoma of the cervix by radiotherapy or surgery should give an 85-90 per cent five-year cure rate; treatment of stage II by radiotherapy about 50-60 per cent; stage III, 35-45 per cent; and stage IV, depending on the selection, a 10-15 per cent five-year cure rate.

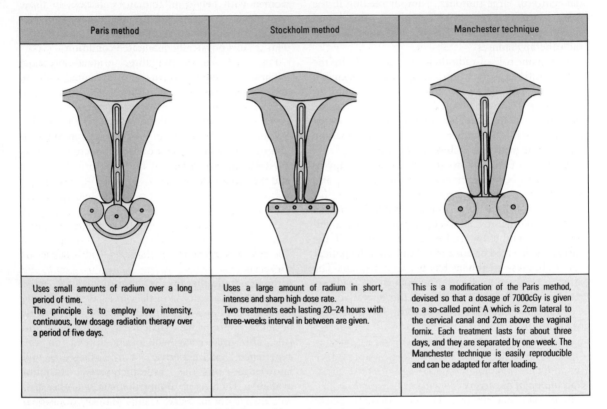

Paris method	Stockholm method	Manchester technique
Uses small amounts of radium over a long period of time. The principle is to employ low intensity, continuous, low dosage radiation therapy over a period of five days.	Uses a large amount of radium in short, intense and sharp high dose rate. Two treatments each lasting 20–24 hours with three-weeks interval in between are given.	This is a modification of the Paris method, devised so that a dosage of 7000cGy is given to a so-called point A which is 2cm lateral to the cervical canal and 2cm above the vaginal fornix. Each treatment lasts for about three days, and they are separated by one week. The Manchester technique is easily reproducible and can be adapted for after loading.

Fig. 10.3 The three original methods of giving intracavity and vaginal radium, for carcinoma of the cervix.

Fig. 10.4 Those factors which may indicate that surgery is preferable to radiotherapy in treatment of carcinoma of the cervix.

SURGERY FOR CARCINOMA OF THE CERVIX STAGE I AND STAGE IIA

Preferable
young, fit, healthy women aged under 40 in whom ovaries may be conserved
*endocervical 'barrel-shaped' carcinomas (or combined therapy)

Associated pathology
presence of large fibroids or ovarian cyst
pelvic inflammatory disease
ulcerative colitis
diverticulitis

Other factors
very narrow vagina, such that is impossible to insert
impossible to identify uterine cavity or cervical canal
unsatisfactory placement of radioactive sources after several attempts

Carcinoma of the endometrium

The prognosis of this cancer depends on three factors:

(i)   The cell type and its differentiation.
(ii) The degrees of myometrial involvement.
(iii) The presence or absence of endocervical involvement.

Adenocarcinoma is the commonest primary tumour, and since it occurs commonly in postmenopausal women it is associated with postmenopausal bleeding. When it occurs in premenopausal women it causes intermenstrual bleeding. These early symptoms are regarded by the woman and her medical attendants as a sign of cancer and the patients therefore present to the general practitioner early and are referred for diagnosis and treatment urgently. Although stage-for-stage, carcinoma of the endometrium and cervix have a similar prognosis, the majority of women (at least 80 per cent) with carcinoma of the endometrium present with Stage I disease, compared with only 20 per cent of those women with carcinoma of the cervix. Whilst the tumour is also likely to be well-differentiated, which improves the prognosis the association of obesity, diabetes and hypertension makes these women a high-risk group.

Primary surgery includes a total abdominal hysterectomy and bilateral salpingo-oophorectomy with the removal of a vaginal cuff, but to some extent the patients will be selected on their fitness for operation. The reported incidence of vaginal recurrence after total hysterectomy varies from ten to 15 per cent and the most common site of recurrence is the vaginal vault. Many gynaecologists will therefore routinely recommend postoperative radiotherapy to the vaginal vault, but, if not routinely, then certainly to those women with moderate or poor differentiation of their tumour and/or if histology confirms involvement of the myometrium.

About one third of the women will be treated with radiotherapy alone because of their associated medical problems or their obesity. Applications of caesium similar to those used for carcinoma of the cervix are then used, but with higher intrauterine dosage. Whole-pelvic irradiation may, as in carcinoma of the cervix, also be used prior to a slightly reduced dosage of intracavity caesium. Indeed, the greater availability of high-energy whole-pelvis irradiation has made this, with a boost from intracavity caesium at the end of the course, the treatment of choice.

Carcinoma of the vagina

The site and extent of the tumour determines the treatment of these tumours, the majority of which will be squamous cell carcinomas. For early lesions in the upper third of the vagina, radiotherapy treatment similar to that for carcinoma of the cervix is given. For advanced stages, the risks of high-dosage radiotherapy often indicate serious consideration of a surgical approach to reduce tumour size and bulk before radiotherapy.

Carcinoma of the vulva

The treatment of choice is surgery. Radiotherapy may be useful as a primary management for those with small localized tumours who refuse surgery or who are medically unfit for surgery. Post-operative therapy is indicated when the resection margins are close to or involved by tumour, and also for those with positive nodes, when the groin should be irradiated.

Carcinoma of the ovary

The role of radiotherapy is only adjuvant as the primary treatment is surgery, the aim being to remove all or as much of the tumour as possible, followed by chemotherapy. The rare malignant germ cell tumours are extremely radiosensitive and radiocurable, and postoperative radiotherapy may be indicated in these cases.

CHEMOTHERAPY

It is acknowledged that some cancers can now be cured by chemotherapeutic agents. The classic example in gynaecology is choriocarcinoma (malignant trophoblastic disease) in which the vast majority of women with metastatic and non-metastatic disease are completely cured by chemotherapy alone. The response of carcinoma of the cervix to the chemotherapy agents available to date is, however, poor and many chemotherapy agents have been tried in ovarian cancer. Although there has been an encouraging response of ovarian tumours to chemotherapy, and significant periods of clinical remission have been noted, few patients are cured. Chemotherapy is now used in the treatment of many gynaecological cancers at an earlier stage in the disease process than previously when it was only considered as a palliative measure.

Both chemotherapy and radiotherapy are dependent on a percentage kill phenomenon; that is, a fixed percentage of the tumour cells will be killed by either technique regardless of the number present at the onset of therapy, and this can influence survival (see Fig. 10.5). Consequently, if there are a large number of tumour cells present or left after surgery, there is, in general, little chance of reducing the number significantly and arresting the progression of the tumour by chemotherapy. An example of this is given in Fig. 10.6. It is important to remember that not all tumour cells will be active at the same time, for if that was the case, then tumour growth would be logarithmic. The rate of tumour growth in fact decreases as a tumour grows, no matter how active it was initially. The amount of time it takes a tumour to double its size increases with increasing bulk. This is because the growth of the tumour

outstrips its blood supply. The centre of most tumours consists of dead or non-dividing cells. The oxygenation of the tissues is also reduced at the centre of a tumour and this partially explains why chemotherapy and radiotherapy are less effective in the presence of bulk disease.

Life cycle of cells

In order to understand chemotherapy of tumours one has to understand the life cycle of the normal and the neoplastic cell. One of the characteristics of tumours is the loss of normal control of cell growth and division. Growth of any tissue is not just a function of the production of cells by mitosis, but the balance between the number of cells which are produced relative to the number that die. So a tumour with a short cell-doubling time and a low rate of cell loss will grow rapidly compared with a tumour with a long cell-doubling time and high rate of cell loss.

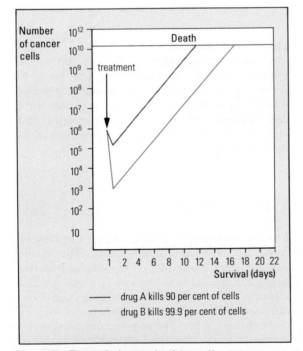

Fig. 10.5 Theoretical example of drug effectiveness. Drug A kills 90 per cent of the tumour cells present at the time of treatment. Drug B is more effective and kills 99.9 per cent of the tumour cells. In this example the host lives five weeks longer when treated with the more effective drug.

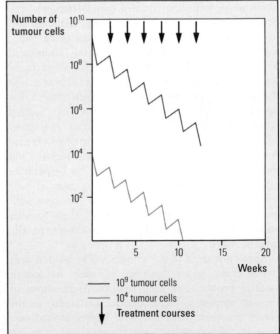

Fig. 10.6 If treatment is initiated with a lower tumour burden, fewer treatment courses are needed and the possibility of drug resistance or prohibitive toxicity is reduced.

Chemotherapeutic agents used for the treatment of malignant tumours vary in their mechanism of action, but they all result in cell death or destruction. This is accomplished by interfering with one or more of the five phases of the cell cycle. These drugs act on all cells, whether normal or malignant, so their toxic action affects normal tissues and cells as well as tumours.

The life cycle of cell division and reproduction of both normal and tumour cells is shown in Fig. 10.7. The cycle begins with cell division (mitosis). After the cell has completed this division it enters the first gap or growth phase (G_1 phase) which is a relatively quiescent phase. During this phase DNA and protein synthesis are initiated. It is the longest phase of the cell cycle and is highly variable in duration and often related to the proliferative activity of the tissue itself. If tissue activity is high, the G_1 phase is short. Occasionally cells rest for prolonged periods and are then known to be in the G_0 phase and during this phase the cell is being primed for DNA synthesis.

After the G_1 phase the cell enters the S phase. During this period, which lasts some ten to 12 hours, the cell doubles its DNA content. Following the S phase there is a premitotic phase (G_2 phase) which lasts from two to ten hours. Finally, there is the mitotic phase (M phase) which lasts 30 to 40 minutes.

It was originally thought that chemotherapeutic drugs might be phase-specific, but this has been proved to not be the case in the case of most agents. Most chemotherapeutic agents act in several phases

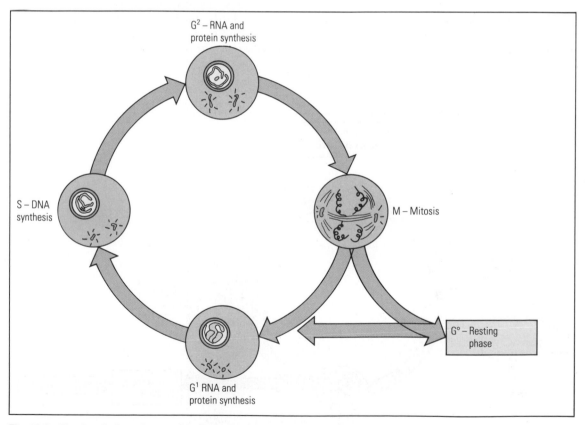

Fig. 10.7 The five distinct phases of the cell cycle begin with mitosis (M). An interval of variable duration follows, during which there is an absence of DNA synthesis and a diploid DNA content of the cell (G_1). RNA and protein synthesis occur during the G_1 phase. If this phase is prolonged, the cell is considered to have entered a resting or non-dividing phase (G_0). DNA synthesis occurs during the S phase in which the entire complement of DNA is duplicated. A second postmitotic gap with no DNA synthesis then occurs (G_2). During the M phase the cell divides into two daughter cells each of which receives a diploid DNA content.

of the cell cycle. Agents which are most effective in the S phase are usually effective inhibitors of rapidly proliferating cell populations. Conversely, alkylating agents and other drugs such as adriamycin seem to be largely independent of the cell reproduction cycle and are effective against tumours displaying relatively low proliferative activity. Some examples of the various chemotherapeutic agents in relation to the phases of the cell cycle are given in Fig. 10.8.

Pharmacology studies

One of the principles of modern anti-cancer chemotherapy is to ensure the maximum therapeutic response and minimum toxicity. Currently no single treatment, whether with one or several drugs, eliminates all the tumour cells of the neoplasm. All anti-cancer drugs kill a constant percentage of the tumour cells.

In order for a tumour to be detected a tumour must have a volume of at least 1ml ($1cm^3$), consisting of about 10^9 cells. The volume of cells necessary to kill a patient is 1000ml ($1000cm^3$), or about 10^{12} (one trillion) cells. Since a given drug kills a constant percentage of cells, and not a constant number of cells, the drug dose and the ability to eradicate cells are related. The major problem is the toxicity of the drug on other tissues. With existing drugs, improved results can only occur if treatment is started before the volume of the tumour is too large. Chemotherapy is therefore rendered more effective following surgical reduction of the tumour mass. In order to maximise the potential for cure by chemotherapy treatment, it should be started as soon as possible after surgery. Combination chemotherapy should also be used for maximal effectiveness.

The introduction of new drugs is a lengthy process and it has to be monitored very precisely, particularly with regard to chemotherapeutic agents which have an effect on normal cells as well as tumour cells. Fig.

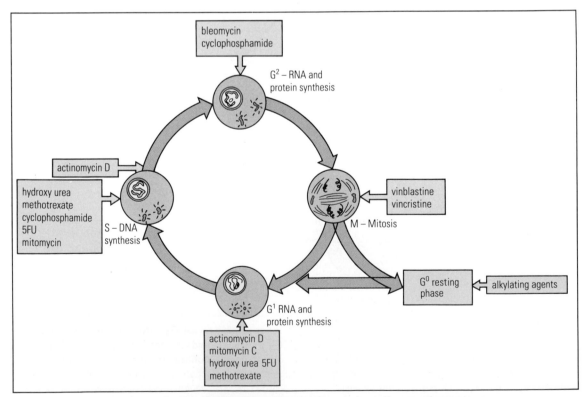

Fig. 10.8 The sites of action on the five phases of the cell cycle of some chemotherapeutic agents.

10.9 outlines the pattern for drug development and Fig. 10.10 the types of clinical trials which always have to be approved by ethical committees.

Chemotherapy regimes

Complete remission is a pre-requisite to achieve cure and significantly prolong survival. Maximum drug dosages must be given in order to achieve maximum killing of tumour cells, since reducing the dose to minimise toxicity may be ineffective, and so of no benefit to the patient.

Combination therapy for most gynaecological cancers is superior to single-agent chemotherapy. Single agents are associated with reduced survival and eventual regrowth of the tumour with resistant tumour cells. Drug therapies should be designed to combine agents which produce different biochemical reactions and so multiple sites of attack in the biosynthetic pathways of cellular function can be achieved. The specific sequence of administering multiple drugs in combination therapy regimes is variable and to some extent dependent on the route of administration for a particular drug. For example, the intravenous route is preferred for water soluble compounds, as complete absorption is guaranteed when the infusion is completed.

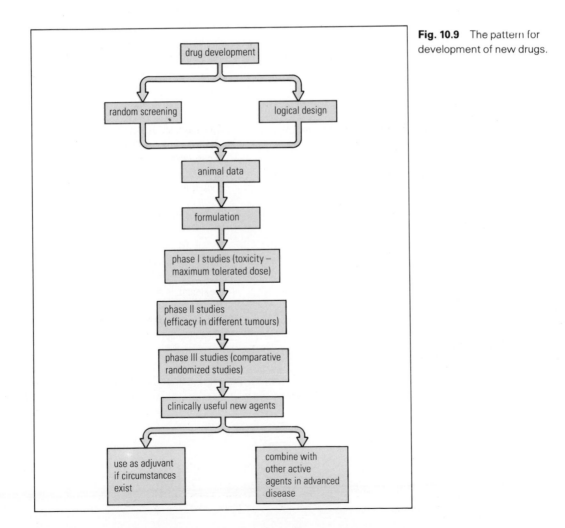

Fig. 10.9 The pattern for development of new drugs.

The chemotherapy of gynaecological cancer has made major progress over the last decade and this is associated with centralisation of treatment, often by specialist medical oncologists. All those treating these patients must understand the effectiveness of chemotherapy and its relationship to surgery and radiotherapy. The goal of all therapy should be disease-free survival, if cure is not possible. The quality of survival is also a major consideration, bearing in mind the effect that all treatments of gynaecological cancer can have on other tissues.

TYPES OF CLINICAL TRIALS		
Phase	Goal	Comment
I	Determine the maximum tolerated dose for a given schedule of a drug in humans	The mechanism of action, likely toxicities, and probable useful schedule are generally available from preclinical animal studies. Patients do not have to have measurable disease for study entry.
II	Define the spectrum of anti-tumour action of a drug	The maximum tolerated dose of drug is used in patients with different kinds of measurable cancer. The response rate is determined and rare side effects are looked for.
III	Compare two or more drugs, drug schedules, or drug combination to define the clinical value of a new therapy more precisely	This is usually conducted as a randomized clinical trial with the control group receiving 'standard' treatment. In some cases, this may include the use of a placebo or the use of supportive care without chemotherapy.

Fig. 10.10 Clinical trials, used in the evaluation of new drugs.

11

Gynaecological Operations

Most gyneacological surgery is performed as a planned procedure on a healthy woman admitted to hospital for surgery. This so-called elective surgery allows time for careful preoperative assessment. On occasions, emergency surgery may be necessary on account of the condition of the patient; ruptured ectopic pregnancy is a good example of such a life-threatening situation requiring emergency surgery.

PREOPERATIVE ASSESSMENT

The preoperative assessment is summarized in Fig. 11.1.

Psychological

It is important that the patient has a clear understanding of the surgery proposed, and of the prognosis and possible complications of the surgery. This is particularly important when the surgery is for a non-life-threatening condition since it is possible that surgery may not resolve the condition or indeed may make it worse (e.g. surgery for urinary incontinence).

Physical

The past history of the patient must be documented carefully. Drug use or allergic reaction must be noted. Use of tobacco or alcohol may affect the risk of anaesthesia and surgery, and the patient should be warned of this.

The general physical condition of the patient should be assessed. The haemoglobin level should be measured and, unless surgery is urgent, deficiency of iron or folic acid should be corrected before surgery. Thyroid disease is not uncommon in women who have heavy menstrual loss and anaemia. A history of easy bruising may reveal a blood-clotting disorder which may be responsible for the menstrual disorder. The breast should be carefully examined for disease. The pulse and blood pressure are measured, and an electrocardiograph recorded when ischaemic heart disease is suggested by the history or examination. Hypertension or heart failure must be treated before surgery is contemplated. Auscultation of the lung fields is important to exclude infection or secondary disease. Respiratory tract infection will be exacerbated by general anaesthesia and should therefore be treated before surgery in non-urgent cases. Abdominal examination is important to demonstrate hepatic enlargement when present. Pelvic surgery

PREOPERATIVE ASSESSMENT FOR GYNAECOLOGICAL SURGERY

psyche

conjunctiva (for anaemia)

thyroid

auscultation of the heart

electrocardiograph

breasts

auscultation of the lung fields

haemoglobin

blood group

urea and electrolytes

cross-match blood

abdominal and pelvic examination

blood pressure and pulse

varicose veins or obesity – consider anti-coagulation

Fig. 11.1 Preoperative assessment for gynaecological surgery.

carries a significant risk of deep vein thrombosis and pulmonary embolism, particularly in obese women who use tobacco. Women should be encouraged to lose weight and stop smoking before surgery, and anti-coagulant prophylaxis is employed by many surgeons on a routine basis to cover major pelvic surgery. Urea and electrolytes must be measured in hypertensive women or women on diuretic therapy. Because of the risk of serious blood loss associated with intermediate and major pelvic surgery, blood is taken at the preoperative assessment for grouping and saving serum or for cross-matching.

GYNAECOLOGICAL OPERATIONS

Endometrial curettage

The operation is performed to determine the contents of the uterine cavity. It is commonly referred to as a 'D and C', which is an abbreviation for dilatation of the cervix and curettage of the uterine cavity. If a small sample of the endometrium is required (to examine the status of the endometrial cells), endometrial biopsy may be performed in the outpatient clinic without anaesthesia using a fine plastic suction curette (Fig. 11.2).

Procedure

The operation is generally performed under general anaesthesia using full aseptic precautions. The patient is placed in the lithotomy position and the bladder is emptied using a urethral catheter so that a full examination of the pelvis can be performed with the patient relaxed and without a distended bladder masking any pelvic masses. A fine uterine sound is passed through the cervix until the tip reaches the uterine fundus, thereby determining the length of the uterine cavity. The cervix is then opened or dilated using dilators of increasing diameter until the cervix is sufficiently open to insert polyp forceps and a curette. The polyp forceps are introduced into the uterine cavity and any polyps are grasped and twisted free from the uterine wall. Cervical polyps can also be removed in this way. The uterus is now

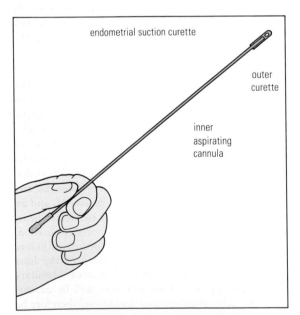

Fig. 11.2 Endometrial biopsy. A small sample of endometrium is curetted and aspirated into the plastic cannula by withdrawal of the central cannula.

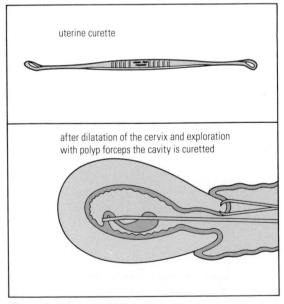

Fig. 11.3 Endometrial curettage.

curetted with a sharp curette (Fig. 11.3) and the sample removed and sent for histological examination.

Endometrial curettage is performed after incomplete miscarriage or with a missed abortion or blighted ovum (see Chapter 5). With termination of pregnancy, the uterus is evacuated with a suction curette after cervical dilatation (Fig. 11.4) which aspirates the uterine contents as they are separated from the uterine wall by curettage.

Complications

Immediate

Perforation of the uterus is the most common complication. In most cases no further action is required, but if there excessive bleeding through the cervix or into the peritoneal cavity, or bowel has been grasped by the polyp forceps, an exploratory laparoscopy or laparotomy may be required. The pregnant uterus is softer and more vascular, and therefore complications are more common when curettage is performed in pregnancy.

Late

The procedure may introduce infection into the pelvis which may lead to damage to the Fallopian tubes. Perforation of the uterus can impair the strength of the uterine wall which has important implications in pregnancy and labour. Over-vigorous curettage in the presence of infection may lead to the formation of intrauterine adhesions which result in oligomenorrhoea and infertility.

Laparoscopy

Laparoscopy involves the introduction of a fibreoptic telescope into the peritoneal cavity to visualize the pelvic viscera. It is particularly valuable as a diagnostic tool in the diagnosis of unexplained pelvic pain, ectopic pregnancy and obstructed Fallopian tubes. It is also used for the occlusion of the Fallopian tubes at sterilization with clips or rings, for the aspiration of ovarian follicles, and for the placement of gametes or zygotes into the Fallopian tubes in assisted reproduction. Other surgical pro-

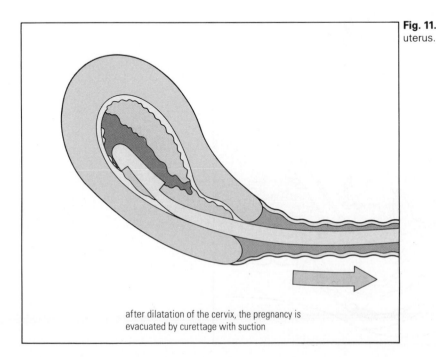

Fig. 11.4 Suction evacuation of the uterus.

after dilatation of the cervix, the pregnancy is evacuated by curettage with suction

cedures, such as diathermy or laser to deposits of endometriosis, plication of the round ligaments (ventrosuspension), and division of adhesions, may be performed with the aid of a laparoscope.

Procedure

The operation is generally performed under general anaesthesia and ventilation is advisable. The patient is placed in a flattened lithotomy position and full aseptic precautions taken. To separate the anterior abdominal wall from the intra-abdominal contents, the abdominal cavity is filled with carbon dioxide through a needle introduced through the anterior abdominal wall and then removed.

The laparoscope is introduced through a cannula which is inserted through the anterior abdominal wall through a subumbilical incision. Unless there are adhesions or large masses, the pelvic viscera and any abnormality within can be clearly visualized. If methylene blue dye is inserted through the cervix, it can normally be seen passing along the Fallopian tubes and spilling from the fimbrial end of the tube. If sterilization is required, the Fallopian tubes may be occluded by a clip ('Filshie clip') applied with an applicator introduced through another small incision (Fig. 11.5).

Complications

Early

The commonest complication is perforation of an intra-abdominal viscus by the carbon-dioxide-insufflating needle or by the laparoscope introducing trochar. If the perforation is recognized, immediate action can be taken to repair the damage. However, damage to bowel, for example, may not be recognized since the insertion of the needle and trochar is blind and the hole in the bowel may not be visible when the laparoscope is introduced. Symptoms and signs of peritonitis after laparoscopy must therefore be regarded with great suspicion.

Late

Laparoscopy may introduce infection into the peritoneal cavity which may result in adhesions which may in turn impair fertility.

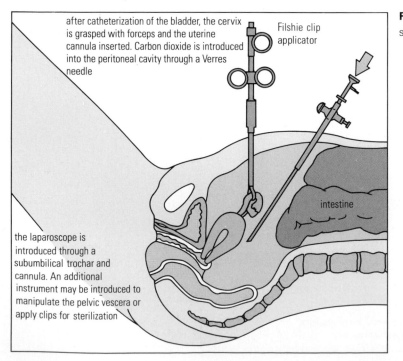

after catheterization of the bladder, the cervix is grasped with forceps and the uterine cannula inserted. Carbon dioxide is introduced into the peritoneal cavity through a Verres needle

Filshie clip applicator

intestine

the laparoscope is introduced through a subumbilical trochar and cannula. An additional instrument may be introduced to manipulate the pelvic viscera or apply clips for sterilization

Fig. 11.5 Laparoscopy and sterilization

Hysteroscopy

The hysteroscope is used to visualize the endometrial cavity (Fig. 11.6). This may be useful where an intrauterine anatomical abnormality is suspected, where intrauterine adhesions may have formed (see above) or for placement of gametes or zygotes into the Fallopian tubes in assisted reproduction. The endometrium is removed under hysteroscopic vision by either laser or resection.

Procedure

The procedure is performed under general anaesthesia with the patient in the lithotomy position. Full aseptic precautions are used. The hysteroscope is introduced through the cervix and the field of vision is kept clear by saline lavage in normal hysteroscopy, or by glycine in endometrial ablation.

Complications

The procedure may introduce infection to the pelvis. Uterine perforation with the hysteroscope or laser is a risk, but the main concern with long hysteroscopic procedures is of lavage fluid overload. In addition, hyponatraemia and glycine encephalopathy have been reported.

Surgery of the cervix

For cervical incompetence, see p.79 for the insertion of a suture.

Small lesions of the cervix such as cervical erosions (ectopy) can be treated by cryotherapy. Cervical intraepithelial neoplasia, providing that the lesion can be totally visualized, can be treated by diathemy, laser therapy or a cold coagulator (Fig. 11.7).

Cone biopsy

Cone biopsy of the cervix may be performed as a diagnostic or therapeutic procedure. When the transformation zone is not fully visualized at colposcopy, cone biopsy is requied to determine the severity of the cervical neoplasia. Cone biopsy may be used to remove intraepithelial neoplasia when a

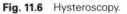

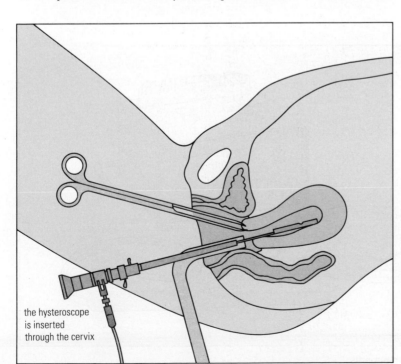

the hysteroscope is inserted through the cervix

Fig. 11.6 Hysteroscopy.

colposcopically-directed biopsy has defined the disease.

Procedure

Traditionally, cone biopsy was performed with a knife (Fig. 11.8), but more recently, laser has been used to excise the cone or ablate the cervical tissue. The procedure is performed under general anaesthesia using full aseptic precautions. After removal of the cone of cervical tissue, the cervix is often oversewn or left open after laser excision.

Complications

Early

The main complication is haemorrhage. This may be substantial and is managed by either packing the vagina or resuturing the wound.

Late

Secondary haemorrhage owing to infection may occur. This may also be substantial and can only be treated by packing the vagina, since the tissues are soft and infected and cannot be sutured. Secondary haemorrhage usually occurs within two weeks of the cone biopsy. Cervical stenosis may be produced by cone biopsy. This may present a few months after operation with amenorrhea and cyclical pelvic pain. Cervical dilatation is required to release the menstrual blood. Cervical stenosis may present in labour when the cervix fails to dilate in the presence of strong uterine contractions. Caesarean section must be performed in such cases to prevent tearing of the cervix. Aternatively, the cervix may be incompetent after cone biopsy and second-trimester miscarriage may result.

Surgery to the Fallopian tubes and ovaries

Surgery to the Fallopian tubes may be either constructive or destructive. Where tubal occlusion is present, either following sterilization or infection, the tube may be made patent by removing the occluded portion and re-anastomosing each side of the occluded parts (Fig. 11.9). Fertility is most likely to be restored if the fimbrial end of the tube is normal and this is most commonly found where pelvic infection has

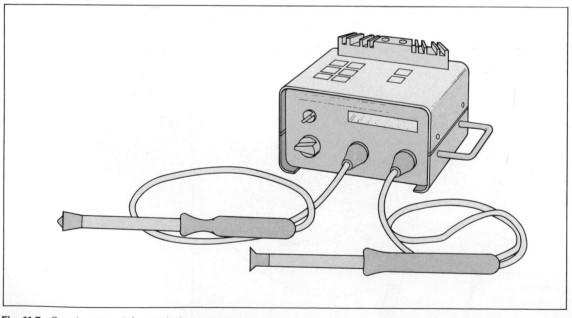

Fig. 11.7 Cryotherapy unit for cervical treatments.

caused sterility by adhesions which separate the fimbrial end of the tube from the ovary. Unfortunately, damage to the endosalpinx is common with pelvic infection so that restoration of tubal patency does not of itself restore normal tubal function. Sterilization may be performed by occluding the tubal lumen with clips, rings, diathermy or by tubal ligation. All methods carry a risk of failure (one in 500) and of ectopic pregnancy. Fallopian tube surgery is most commonly performed as an emergency when there is an ectopic pregnancy in the tube. If the tube has ruptured salpingectomy is necessary. The tube may be conserved if rupture has not occurred; the tube is opened, the pregnancy removed and the tube reconstituted. The risk of recurrent ectopic pregnancy in such cases is high.

Surgery to the ovaries is either conservative or radical. Where possible, ovarian tissue is conserved and the cyst or endometriotic deposits are separated from the ovary (ovarian cystectomy). Wedge resection of the ovary is now carried out less frequently than previously, because of the successful medical management of polycystic ovarian disease and the risk of iatrogenic tubal adhesion. If there is no healthy ovarian tissue remaining or if malignancy if found, oophorectomy is performed.

Complications
Early
The Fallopian tubes and ovaries are vascular structures and careful haemostasis is required at surgery. Inadequate ligature of pedicles at such surgery can result in massive intraperitoneal haemorrhage.

Late
Adhesions following surgery to the tubes and ovaries are common and may impair fertility.

Uterine surgery

Conservative
The most common conservative uterine surgery is myomectomy or removal of uterine fibroids in a woman who wishes to retain her uterus (usually to

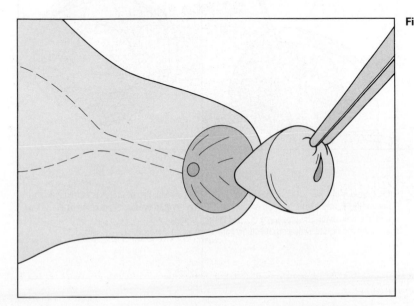

Fig. 11.8 Cone biopsy of the cervix.

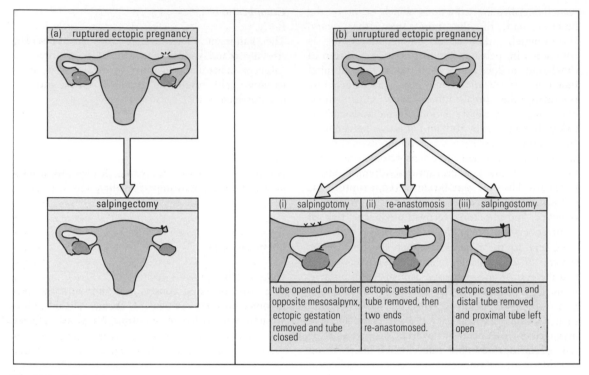

Fig. 11.9 Tubal surgery.

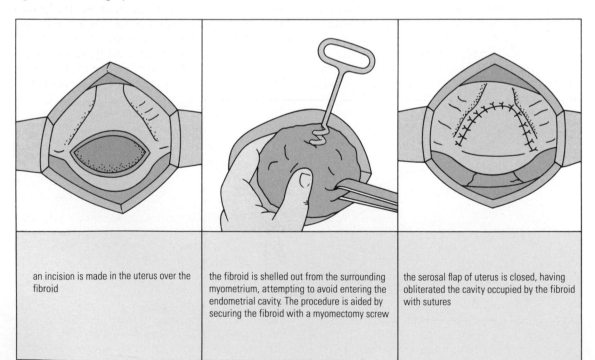

Fig. 11.10 Myomectomy.

have more children). Fibroids are often large and multiple, and surgery can involve considerable blood loss. In principle, when removing the fibroids the aim is to minimize the damage to the serosal surface of the uterus and to try to avoid opening the uterine cavity (Fig. 11.10). The morbidity following myomectomy is no less than that following hysterectomy and women who require fibroid removal are therefore encouraged to have a hysterectomy unless they wish to extend their family. Conservative surgery to correct congenital anatomical defects is occasionally performed in women who have a history of recurrent miscarriage (Fig. 11.11).

Total

Hysterectomy is most commonly performed in women who have begnign conditions which produce menstrual disorder. In most cases the cervix is removed with the uterus (total hysterectomy), but occasionally, because of technical difficulty, the cervix may be retained (subtotal hysterectomy). The ovaries are normally conserved at hysterectomy but in older women the risk of developing ovarian carcinoma may be judged to be higher than the benefit from ovarian conservation. The ovaries are removed when endometrial carcinoma is present. In radical hysterectomy (Wertheim's hysterectomy) for carcinoma of the cervix, the pelvic lymph nodes are also removed but the ovaries are normally conserved. This confers an advantage of surgery over radiotherapy for treatment of cervical carcinoma, since radiotherapy causes loss of ovarian function.

Hysterectomy may be performed abdominally or vaginally. If the uterus is large, there is a history of pelvic infection, there is minimal uterine prolapse, the subpubic arch is narrow, or there is a suspicion of malignancy, the uterus is normally removed abdominally (Fig. 11.12).

Procedure
Abdominal hysterectomy

General anaesthesia is usually used. The operation is generally performed through a low transverse incision (Fig. 11.13). Three clamps on either side of the uterus are usually required to occlude the blood supply from the ovarian, uterine and vaginal blood vessels. The vagina is cut around the cervix and closed so that it becomes a blind-ending pouch. The bladder must be dissected free from the cervix before the cervix can be removed. After caesarean section or cone biopsy, the bladder may be more adherent to the cervix and additional care is needed to avoid bladder injury. The ureters pass close to the lateral fornices of the vagina and this is the most common site for ureteric injury during hysterectomy.

Vaginal hysterectomy

Vaginal hysterectomy is the method of choice for removal of the uterus in a parous woman whose uterus is not larger than a 12-week size pregnancy. In principle, removal of the uterus is the same as in abdominal hysterectomy, but, with the vaginal route, the first clamp is applied at the bottom of the uterus on the cardinal and uterosacral ligaments. To the patient there is the considerable advantage that there is no painful abdominal wound. Technically, vaginal hysterectomy may be more difficult because of the limited access through the vagina, and is therefore less popular with some gynaecologists. When there is vaginal prolapse this can be repaired at the same time as vaginal hysterectomy. Cystocele (see Chapter 6) is repaired by dissection of the bladder from the anterior vaginal wall and support of the bladder with a layer of fascia (pubocervical fascia) under the bladder base. Similarly, rectocele is repaired by dissection of the rectum from the posterior vaginal wall and suture of the fascia overlying the levator ani in front of the rectum, so preventing descent. If an enterocele is present, the peritoneal sac must be fully defined and the uterosacral ligaments drawn together to occlude the lumen of the sac.

Complications
Early

The most common complication immediately after hysterectomy is haemorrhage. If the haemorrhage is intraperitoneal, the early warning will be tachycardia and hypotension which will eventually be followed by abdominal distension and pain. However, considerable blood loss occurs before abdominal distension is obvious, and pain is normal immediately after surgery. Vaginal bleeding after hysterectomy may be stopped with a firm vaginal pack but it is often wiser to identify and arrest the source of bleeding which is usually a vessel at the lateral angle of the vaginal vault.

181

Late

Accumulation of blood at the vaginal vault after hysterectomy can lead to a vault haematoma which will eventually become infected and produce a vault abscess. Vault abscess and urinary tract infection are the commonest causes of febrile morbidity after hysterectomy, and since both occur relatively frequently some surgeons use preoperative or postoperative antibiotic prophylaxis in all women undergoing major surgery. Many women carry pathogenic bacteria in their vagina which predisposes to vault abscess after major surgery.

Dyspareunia is not uncommon after prolapse repair, particularly that which involves the posterior vaginal wall. Women and their partners should be warned about this before surgery and questioned about it on review after surgery.

The introduction of endometrial ablation (see p.177) may reduce the frequency of hysterectomy and the attendant complication of major pelvic surgery. As it becomes a more popular alternative, more complications become apparent so it will be some time before its long-term value can be assessed.

POSTOPERATIVE

First 24 hours

After surgery, patients will usually be transferred to a recovery area. In the recovery area, pulse, blood pressure, respiratory rate and level of consciousness are documented every 5-10 minutes. When the observations are stable for 30-60 minutes, the patient is transferred to the ward. If there are changes in any of these parameters, the cause must be determined. A drop in blood pressure with slow pulse is found in response to atropine-like drugs used in the reversal of paralysis. If this hypotension is caused by hypovolaemia owing to blood loss, there will be a tachycardia and evidence of intraperitoneal or vaginal haemorrhage must be sought (Fig. 11.14). If the patient has not passed urine within six hours of surgery, the abdomen should be examined to see if there is suprapubic distension because of urinary retention. Catheterization is necessary if the patient is unable to pass urine.

One day to six days

After 24 hours (in many cases before), most minor and intermediate gynaecological surgery cases will be fit for discharge. Before discharge, the patient must be fully conscious and orientated. Pulse and blood pressure should be unchanged from the preoperative state. The abdomen should be soft and not unduly tender. No new masses should be palpable and bowel sounds should be audible. After laparoscopy, it is common for women to have some mild abdominal tenderness and shoulder discomfort (referred from diaphragmatic irritation by carbon dioxide in-

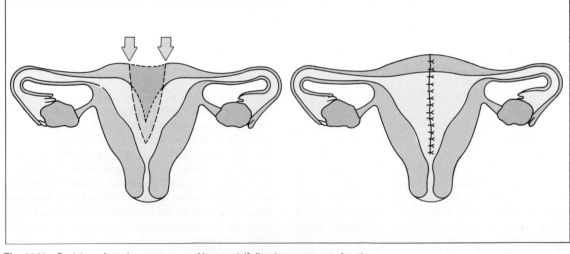

Fig. 11.11 Excision of uterine septum and its repair following recurrent abortion.

sufflation), but they should be apyrexial and bowel sounds should be audible. Vaginal bleeding after endometrial curettage should be no worse than normal menstrual loss. After major pelvic surgery some intestinal ileus is common. If bowel sounds have not resumed, oral intake should be restricted and an intravenous infusion maintained. An indwelling catheter may be necessary for a few days to prevent urinary retention, particularly after prolapse repair. The patient should be examined daily and more frequently if there are problems. The chest should be examined for signs of infection and physiotherapy prescribed if expectoration is difficult and infection suspected. If there is a pyrexia, the site of infection must be determined. Infection of the abdominal or vaginal wound will lead to swinging pyrexia with the temperature being elevated at night. Urinary infection will generally produce a continuous pyrexia. The legs must be examined regularly for evidence of deep vein thrombosis.

Patients who have undergone major pelvic surgery will usually be mobilized quickly since this is important in prevention of venous thrombosis, and discharge will normally be encouraged within one week. Postoperative complications will lengthen the period of hospitalization and all patients must be apyrexial, and must be able to empty bowel and bladder normally on discharge. Women who have had a prolapse repair must have a vaginal examination before discharge from hospital to break down any adhesions between anterior and posterior vaginal wall wounds.

INDICATIONS FOR VAGINAL HYSTERECTOMY

1. Patient comfort/convenience
   There is no abdominal wound so postoperative period is more comfortable

2. Uterus less than size of 12-week pregnancy
   Larger uterus can be removed vaginally, but technical difficulty increases with uterine size

3. Uterine and/or vaginal prolapse
   Uterus is easier to remove when there is prolapse. Note: there may be considerable elongation of the cervix without much descent of the uterine body. When vaginal prolapse is present the uterus should be removed vaginally.

4. Subpubic arch
   A narrow subpubic arch makes vaginal surgery more difficult
   wide arch good visibility and access
   narrow arch poor visibility and access

5. Past history of pelvic pain or infection
   A thorough examination of the pelvic viscera cannot be performed at vaginal hysterectomy, so a past history of pain or infection should direct to abdominal surgery. Infection may also produce adhesions which are better approached through abdominal incision.

Fig. 11.12   Indications for vaginal hysterectomy.

Seven days to four weeks

After major surgery, most women are surprised at how tired they become with minimal exertion on returning home. They should be warned of this and should not travel long distances because of the potential risk of secondary haemorrhage owing to vaginal vault infection. During the first two weeks at home they should gradually increase their exercise, aiming at more normal routines after about a month; however, older women may take longer. Intercourse is generally not advisable within this period and the patient is also advised not to drive.

Four weeks onwards

The patient can resume normal activity unless there have been complications. Women who have had a prolapse repair should avoid any heavy lifting for 2–3 months to allow fibrosis to be completed without tissues strain. Women are generally reviewed about six weeks after discharge from hospital, when most will be ready to return to work and resume a normal life. Vaginal discharge from granulation tissue on the vaginal wound is a common complaint but may be resolved by silver nitrate cauterization in the clinic. It is important to examine women who have had a prolapse repair to ensure a satisfactory repair and that there are no adhesions between anterior and posterior vaginal wall wounds.

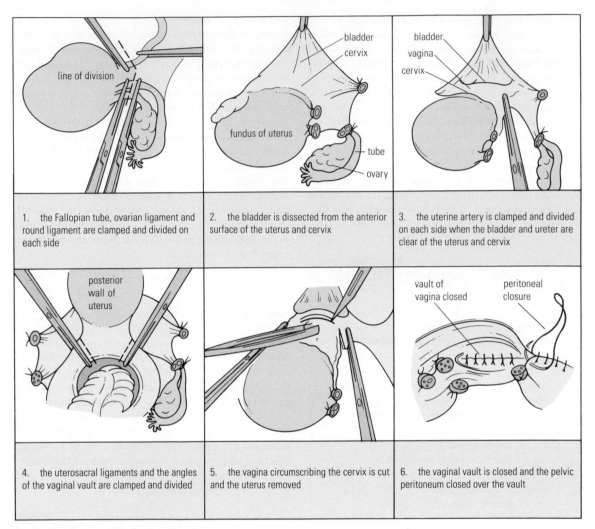

1. the Fallopian tube, ovarian ligament and round ligament are clamped and divided on each side

2. the bladder is dissected from the anterior surface of the uterus and cervix

3. the uterine artery is clamped and divided on each side when the bladder and ureter are clear of the uterus and cervix

4. the uterosacral ligaments and the angles of the vaginal vault are clamped and divided

5. the vagina circumscribing the cervix is cut and the uterus removed

6. the vaginal vault is closed and the pelvic peritoneum closed over the vault

Fig. 11.13 Total abdominal hysterectomy.

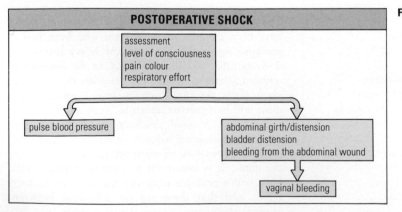

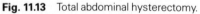

Fig. 11.14 Postoperative shock.

Index